Reflections *on* Health

IN OUR NAKEDNESS, WHO ARE WE?

WRITTEN BY **BRYAN HALE** DC

CHIROPRACTOR

ISBN 978-0-473-40331-7

Published in New Zealand in 2017 by
Hale Technique Publishing Ltd.
149 Barrington Street
Somerfield, Christchurch 8024

Designed and printed by
CAXTON
www.caxton.co.nz

Contents

Acknowledgements   5

Foreword   7

About Bryan   9

Childhood experiences   11

Integrated Health   15

The Hale Technique   17

Early case histories   25

Clearer picture   31

Body-Mind balance   35

Key influences   37

How the Hale Technique works   41

Treatment protocol   45

Beliefs   51

Instincts   53

Values   55

Emotions   57

Key emotions "I feel"   73

Emotions (Key, Supportive, Complex)   75

Emotional/Mental chart   135

The mental mind "I think"   137

Depression/anxiety/melancholy   157

Stress   171

Fear of success   175

Spiritual side   179

Your life purpose   195

Leadership   207

Forgiveness   213

In conclusion (as a practitioner)   225

In conclusion (as Bryan)   229

Bibliography   233

Areas of the body associated with emotional imbalance . . .   234

Index   236

DEDICATIONS

This book is dedicated to my patients, and the Universe;
they have been my great teachers. It is dedicated also to
my dear wife Joanne, my children Belinda and Matthew,
my mentor and great friend Maureen Rose, my Mum, Dad, and
sister Julie-Anne – all great teachers too. I dedicate
this work to you, my readers, as well – in the hope that
you are helped in some way by these words.

Acknowledgements

*"I acknowledge the Universe, my family, my friends, my patients,
and my mentors. They have all challenged me to make choices
that, in turn, may help others heal themselves by firstly
accepting their own behaviour, then understanding others
and themselves, thereby promoting healing and
growth through forgiveness."*
(Bryan Hale)

This book would never have happened without a number of people, for whom I am most grateful. My wife Joanne for her patience, my daughter Belinda for her support, my niece Fiona for reading those early drafts, my mentor Maureen Rose who helped me realise my true purpose and showed me the way, my associates for their encouragement, and my many friends and colleagues over the years. It would never have happened either were it not for my Mum, my sister, and my Dad.

I cannot thank enough my insightful and ingenious editor, Sorcha O'Malley; she worked closely with me, ensuring that my words were clearly expressed as well as true to my own voice. In return, I treated her so effectively that she changed from subservient to bossy!

I would also like to acknowledge the Thursday Night Cashmere Tennis Club Boys for their behaviour, friendship, teachings, and tolerance over the last thirty years. A men-only group, aged between forty-five years and mid-eighties who meet weekly, play tennis, have a couple of drinks, and eat a meal prepared by the member who has been nominated to do so that week.

Men talk and behave very differently to the opposite sex, especially when they are in a male-only group. Sport is the drawcard and I've observed that men who have played team sports cope better with the banter than those who only played individual sports when growing up. Tennis is the physical endeavour, but after that there are emotional and mental challenges for all present when the group becomes a melting pot of jokes, stories, and a lot of embellishment of the facts. This behaviour has intrigued me and taught me a lot about men – in particular concerning their lives, beliefs, values, etc. A few tears are shed and fellow comforting goes on when we have lost good members of our group, but mainly Thursday nights consist of comradery, laughter, and general hilarity.

I sit, observe, and learn. Every now and then I and others try to introduce some controversy into the conversation to keep the dialogue alive and impromptu. We all come from different walks of life, professions, trades, and relationship backgrounds. We are a great group of friends, mates, and 'fri-mates' (combination of a friend and a mate). Very rarely do we learn anything that is worth repeating or useful to know; men relaxing and being able to speak freely amongst themselves without fear of it spreading further is what it's all about.

Thank you to all who have participated in the past and to those who continue to attend most Thursdays.

Thank you to everyone who has taught me something on my journey.

Bryan Hale
Chiropractor

Foreword

The uniqueness of the Hale Technique lies in addressing physical ailments by evaluating a patient's physical, emotional, mental, and spiritual energy state (referred to as 'PEMS' from this point on), and then treatment with gentle chiropractic, homeopathic, and energy-balancing techniques. My practice offers an original approach to health, formulated over more than thirty years of testing – mostly on my patients – gathering patient feedback and combining different health disciplines.

A practitioner can balance the emotional, physical, and spiritual energies. But in order to alter thinking – the mental – a patient must be challenged. This is where we find the most resistance. A patient who accepts a challenge to their thinking is more likely to find acceptance, understanding, and forgiveness. This formula promotes better behaviour; the result is that patients enjoy better physical health.

As a matter of course, all patients must undergo clinical examinations with us to eliminate the possibility of physical disease. Many patients have already had multiple tests, scans, and clinician visits with no real change to their symptoms and conditions. This is when it is time to look deeper.

I started with a belief system that I could influence their health by treating the body structure. Despite being very successful, I wasn't happy with the results I was getting. I realised that there had to be something more to the full health picture. Today, while I'm still first and foremost a chiropractor (a primary healthcare practitioner), I always like to further explore what causes ill health and disease.

The beauty of the Hale Technique is that the further I learn and develop, the more I observe the influence and power of the spiritual/emotional energies that give us direction and learning in this lifetime. The things that challenge us are actually the things we are here to learn.

In this book, I talk about how I see a belief as being neither right nor wrong, good nor bad; nor is it finite. However, issues evolve when beliefs generate negative behaviour patterns.

"Out beyond ideas of wrongdoing and rightdoing,
there is a field. I'll meet you there."
(Rumi)

I hope you take from this book a greater understanding of our authentic selves, our purpose in life, and what our bodies are trying to tell us regarding what we are here to experience and own as a human being.

"If everything were to be taken away from us –
job, house, car, possessions, status – who are we then?
In our nakedness, who are we?"
(Bryan Hale)

About Bryan

Originally, I had intended to be a civil engineer and it was twelve months into this path that I visited my chiropractor, Brian O'Hagan, for pain around my rib cage. He diagnosed that I had early symptoms of shingles. Brian had known me for several years. He explained that shingles was associated with high stress levels and queried if instead of following a career in engineering had I ever considered becoming a chiropractor? That visit changed the course of my life.

When I reported this development to my Mum she was overjoyed as to her it was second best to my becoming a priest! The most relief she had ever received from her chronic health issues was chiropractic treatment. During my childhood, we'd travel to visit a chiropractor only infrequently as every aspect of each trip had to be saved for.

Over the next eighteen months I worked multiple hours in varying jobs so as to save enough money to start studying in Toronto, Canada. After four years of full-time study there I graduated with a Doctor of Chiropractic qualification in 1974.

I am married to Joanne and we have two children and six grandchildren.

My work aside, I'm a typical 'alpha Kiwi male' who enjoys physical fitness and sports, along with an interest in home handyman projects. My favourite spectator sports are rugby union, boxing, ice hockey, and tennis.

I am lucky to have always had a passion for my work. My purpose now is to continue to find out how the body works and help people to learn, grow, heal, find out who they really are, and why they are here in this lifetime.

There is no better fulfilment in life than to have knowledge and to be able to share it.

CHAPTER 1

Childhood experiences formed the basis of my early learning

I was born in February 1949, into my family of my Mum, my Dad, and my sister, Julie-Anne, who is eighteen months older than me. We lived in a two-bedroomed house located in the lower socio-economic area of our small town, Westport, with a population somewhere between four and five thousand people. The economics of the town were based on coal mining, fishing from a local port, and timber. People were hard-working and largely held to good small-town values and pride.

My Mum worked full-time at a chartered accountant's office. She was a very talented person musically and socially, always helping others with arranging concerts, social events, and fundraising gatherings for the church and wider community. Unfortunately for her, health was a major issue. She experienced chronic digestive and bowel issues along with chronic neck and lower back pain. To add to this, she experienced migraine headaches on a weekly basis, only in the weekends, conveniently not causing her any time off work. She was constantly under stress and did not sleep well; she spent her nights reading five to six library books per week (her escape from reality).

When I was three-years-old my Mum was admitted to hospital and put in a plaster cast from her neck to her knees for six months – in an effort to correct the chronic back pain. Julie-Anne was adopted out to another family, but because of my behavioural issues as well as my asthma, eczema, and digestive problems, I stayed home with my Dad. We children managed to see our Mum once per month from the outside fence of the hospital, which was approximately 50m away from the hospital window. The scenario was again repeated when I was seven, but this time my Dad's mother moved in to keep house. To my knowledge, my mother's health pattern never changed until my father passed away when I was sixteen.

My Dad was a very complex person, totally illiterate to the day he died. Because of his difficulties, he left school at age twelve and went to work as a deckhand on the coastal ships that were supplying coal throughout New Zealand. Later he worked on and off as a casual fisherman and on the local wharf as a labourer. He was a very strong man who prided himself on his appearance with regards to his clothing and grooming. Although he was hard-working he never had a full-time paying job until the last four years of his life. As a result, my mother needed to earn enough to keep the family together financially.

Prejudice, biased beliefs and attitudes were his forte. If you disagreed or stood up to him you got punched in the head, unless you were clergy. They could do no wrong, and in their eyes, he could do no wrong either. He (and therefore we as a family) experienced extreme mood swings with resultant bad behaviour. Not only was he violent but one of his main ploys was to not speak to anyone at home for three days, just because his dinner was not on the table at exactly 5.45pm or our bikes were not put away tidily. Outside the house, you could not shut him up when talking to the few people he chose to communicate with. He was an angel outside the home and most people saw him as being a holy, pious man as he went to Mass (church service) every morning and was always helping the nuns and priests with their work. He had converted to Catholicism in his mid-thirties just before meeting and marrying my Mum.

To add to his bipolar behaviour, he was also confused about his sexuality. Living with him was a nightmare as he confused love with the need to protect – not just me, but animals also. He could exhibit overcaring, loving behaviour one minute, but extreme anger and violence the next; this sometimes led to animals dying.

It was his choice that Julie-Anne slept with my mother in one bedroom and I slept with him in the other. Needless to say, I experienced all forms of abuse throughout my childhood – from age three until the age of eleven –

when I was finally taken to a psychiatrist who recommended that my father and I be separated.

Throughout my childhood, I was a very troubled and often violent child who physically fought not only with children of any age in my neighbourhood, but also with their parents, and with the nuns who tried to teach me at school. The nuns were Irish Catholic and were very often harsh and cruel. They often told me, "You have the face of an angel but the devil lives in your heart." They did their very best to beat it out of me! I admit my behaviour and attitude was bad, attracting frequent trouble/punishments.

I finally learned to read and write at age eleven. Two years later, after sitting high school entrance exams, I found myself at boarding school, trying to catch up on English and also learn Latin and French! Two months after my fifteenth birthday I negotiated leaving school and going to work. My mother was heartbroken. I started work back home as a postman delivering mail.

My father passed away suddenly when I was sixteen. He had no insurance or savings to cover the cost of his burial, which left the family compromised. My Mum and I had to go to a family friend to ask for money. Fortunately, this friend donated the money, for which I am extremely grateful. However, that day I made a vow to myself, "I will never have money problems in my life."

Soon after that I got promoted to a clerical position (senior supervisor of personnel) in a large city. Some of my staff had university degrees. I had no qualifications, having left high school at the beginning of my third year. At that time sport and alcohol were my two outlets. Unfortunately, at age eighteen I messed up big time. No one was hurt or defamed but me. The only reconciliation my Mum would accept was that I go back to high school to finish my education. In her words, "Education is your ticket to freedom."

I completed high school a year and a half later, during which time, whilst working part-time in all kinds of jobs, I had paid off a replacement car for my Mum. My employer had kept my job open and wanted me to assume my position again. They wanted to sponsor me to go to university for several years to complete further studies relating to my position/job. I chose engineering instead.

In our family, I became the protector of my Mum and sister against my Dad. I was the 'fall guy' by picking up on his mood from a distance and then clowning around until he broke out at me. To my knowledge, he never hit Mum or my sister and my sister was never aware of him hitting our Mum either.

We all struggled. Julie-Anne left home as soon as she completed high school and struggled with anorexia in her teenage years but is good now. We have become very close over latter years and can now talk openly about our childhood years with laughter. Today it seems like an unreal nightmare.

I have done many years of varying therapies, which have assisted me in developing techniques in my work. Through my education in extreme behaviours, illness, and victimhood there is not much that I have not seen or experienced in life.

I now thank the Universe and every one of my teachers and mentors throughout my journey of experiencing and learning about my life as it was.

CHAPTER 2

Integrated Health

B ased in Christchurch, Integrated Health has more than five thousand current patients and over the last thirty years has treated more than thirty thousand patients.

All practitioners come to Integrated Health specifically to learn and use the Hale Technique. I'm very proud of our team who are all conscientious practitioners.

Integrated Health does not advertise. All patients come through personal referral, perhaps the greatest testimonial possible. (Feel better; tell others.)

We are primary healthcare practitioners using Applied Kinesiology as one of the tools we utilise for communication and assessment purposes. Homeopathy in treatment is also a crucial element of our approach.

While regular medicine is most effective for crisis care and serious disease we have found homeopathy effective for functional health problems – disease or imbalance from pushing our bodies too hard (stress). Symptoms like digestive problems, sleep disorders, low energy, depression, anxiety, neck pain, back pain, headaches, allergies, skin problems, flu-like symptoms, respiratory problems, hay fever, sinus problems, chronic infections (for example thrush or cold sores), and emotional fragility can be signs of functional illness.

The human body entity is a clever system with an innate ability to heal itself, but when it is unable to do so, it will present symptoms as a warning signal that something is amiss.

Most of our patients have tried orthodox or mainstream medicine before visiting us. Through experience we observe that not everything has been investigated until the mental and emotional aspects of the mind have been considered.

The approach in our clinic is a combination of:

- The Hale Technique (evaluation and balancing of physical, emotional, mental, and spiritual energies – PEMS)
- Applied Kinesiology (muscle testing and evaluation)
- Complex homeopathy preparations
- Cranial corrections
- Nutritional supplements
- Gentle adjustments of the spine and extremities
- Other procedures to promote wellness and health
- Personal health promotion and advice.

Our mental (thinking) mind is the strongest asset we possess, but it can also be our worst enemy and saboteur. Functional illness comes from the inability of the body to adapt to the extremes of the mental mind, which can cause imbalance of the PEMS[1]. We are the product of genetics, family beliefs and values along with environmental factors (recorded in our physical, emotional, and spiritual systems). As we go through life with all its challenges, these three systems can either grow and adapt to the mental mind or become stuck, resulting in **Dis-ease**.

We often hear people remark that someone is being overly emotional, but the public display of the said emotion is brought about by the interplay of the mental mind interpreting that emotion. For example, during prize-giving ceremonies, weddings, funerals, graduations, personal confrontations, reunions, etc. – where the mental mind analyses the emotion into "What if", "If only", "I wish", etc.

---

1   *'PEMS' refers to the Physical, Emotional, Mental, and Spiritual energies.*

CHAPTER 3

The Hale Technique

The Hale Technique began out of desperation.

Stressed, mentally on a knife's edge, and struggling to recover physically after three car accidents in six months, I had been rebuilding my fitness until I went over on my left ankle playing squash – badly enough to lose consciousness.

My fractured ankle was a life-changing event as my whole health started to deteriorate over the next twelve months. I gained 30kgs (weighing in at 120kgs) and my asthma, hay fever, and environmental allergies all returned with a vengeance.

My digestion also deteriorated to form ulcerative colitis, plus I developed multiple food allergies/intolerances. I could only eat selected steamed vegetables, fresh fish, and brown rice. I was extremely exhausted and very depressed, although in denial about the latter.

Exhaustion meant I was only working two days a week. My body wanted to rest and sleep but I was not recovering. I felt like a burden to my family.

Peculiarly, there was a recurring experience that happened daily where I felt like I was losing consciousness and then travelling down a long tunnel back to my childhood and beyond. Every time this happened I felt a bit better physically – as if my body was trying to heal itself. It was the first clue that healing the present began with dealing with the past.

I sought help from medical and alternative practitioners. Patients also tried to offer advice and referrals. I wasn't ready to accept many of them.

Standard blood tests in those days offered no clues although alternative testing showed high mercury and lead levels, so I had all my amalgam fillings removed and replaced with composite. There probably isn't anything I didn't try and around this time I started using Applied Kinesiology – testing for muscle responses – on myself (self-testing). This marked the very early beginnings of what would become the Hale Technique.

The technique came about through my own intuition. Over time through using 'self-muscle-testing' I was able to transfer this testing to my patients, asking multiple questions without causing them muscle fatigue. This made testing faster and more effective, resulting in better results in less time.

Today the Hale Technique has been mastered by my associates. I now use muscle testing as a language that I can use to ask the body what it needs in order to heal and grow.

Initially I was dismissive because of my beliefs, but results were evident enough that I could not deny what was happening through experimentation. My energy very slowly returned but my allergies and general lack of wellness never changed until many years later.

We had decided to return to New Zealand from Canada and financially I was able to concentrate on putting more time into my family and my own learning.

I had a lot of work to do, theories to prove, and experiments to perform. I was initially interested in chronic structural problems, cranial jaw problems, food and environmental allergies, heavy metal toxicity, farm chemical and environmental toxicity as I knew these could be causing problems – mine and my patients'.

Learning 'self-muscle-testing' was a real advantage as it was fast, and questions can/could push the boundaries on any topic because patients' personalities are eliminated – you ask the body, not the person.

It is important to note that the body will not reveal or answer questions that the person does not want you to know or is hiding. Although it is difficult, there may in some instances be ways around it, i.e. with suspected addiction the body will say no to the word "addiction" because the patient is in denial, however if you ask about "habits" on a scale of one to ten, anything over a five indicates the possibility of out of control addiction issues. The patient does not want you to know, but the word "habits" is identifiable with the body and so information will be revealed.

Because I was frustrated with my own health I chose to investigate the immune system, in particular its response to toxic substances that resulted in allergy-type conditions.

I accumulated relevant foods, chemicals, pollens, antigens and other nasties, but it became impractical to keep them in the office for testing because of personal exposure risk. I was able to purchase most of these in homeopathic nosode form – homeopathic formulas made up from diseased tissue, fungi, viruses, bacteria, parasites, and chemicals. I already had some knowledge and personal experience with homeopathy so my interest in this fascinating field was rekindled.

In my Christchurch practice, I concentrated on structural problems with an emphasis on cranial (skull) and TMJ (jaw) imbalances, and their effects on the spine and pelvis. I worked in conjunction with several dentists who specialised in mouth splints. I found this rewarding and interesting but what I observed was that while patients' conditions stabilised, their healing only ever reached a certain level (holding pattern). This led me to question what other possibilities might be out there.

I started checking patients for allergy/toxicity possibilities as I knew that the immune system was a major contributing factor involved in their health picture. If there appeared to be an issue I talked to that patient to see if they wanted to investigate further. Most did as usually their health was being compromised in some way.

I was convinced, like many other practitioners worldwide, that chemical toxicity was a major global problem, not only at an acute level, but also at a subtler underlying level. Farmers and agricultural workers were directly affected, but was the general public also at risk?

Muscle testing allowed me to develop techniques and homeopathic remedies to address these findings. To begin with I had mixed success, but obviously, there was a lot of interest as I ended up with more than one hundred new patients on a waiting list. Combining this method with elimination diets

I had success at various levels helping patients with food allergy/intolerance, chemical toxicity, chronic fatigue, digestive problems, and also spinal/joint/muscle/bone problems.

Homeopathy appeared to work well so I ordered every nosode[1] available. When I combined these into treatments we gained surprising improvements in the general health of patients. There was always something new and exciting happening but I was still not convinced; I still had a lot to learn.

In this book, I speak from a practitioner's viewpoint. Therefore, I speak from how it appears the body works with regards to the integration of the various fascinating components that influence our behaviour as a human being. In contrast, I do not offer any answers as to how to cure cancer, heart disease, major health conditions or the various forms of mental illnesses. However, through learning and understanding more about what I have learned myself, the reader may take more ownership of their life, health, and welfare, therefore creating a better life for themselves, their families, their friends, and their immediate world.

Two issues bring patients to doctors:

1. Pain and discomfort
2. Fear of loss to physical and mental health in various forms.

Treating symptoms moves patients into a holding pattern of temporary relief without looking at what may have caused the problem originally.

In my observation, health practitioners generally do not teach patients to change by challenging their beliefs. In my early practice, I was pleased when a sufferer found relief but I was frustrated that I most often could not identify what caused the problem. Why is the body unable to respond in the same way that the average cut or bruise is able to heal itself?

As a chiropractor, back and neck pain can be used as an example. Often what was touted as being the activity that caused the pain was an activity that the sufferer had performed many times before without trouble. However, this time they were compromised to a point that it became a chronic weakness or condition for which they sought treatment.

---

1   *Nosodes are homeopathic formulas made up from diseased tissue, fungi, viruses, bacteria, parasites, and chemicals.*

Examination, x-rays, and tests often show that they have chronic degeneration (osteoarthritis) in the area but numerous studies show that the level of joint degeneration does not necessarily correspond to the level of pain/disability.

Doctors/health practitioners often use the experience of pain to later promote the fear of loss and function, thus maintaining a thriving symbiotic relationship of the patient needing the doctor and the doctor needing the patient – with neither of them learning nor moving on.

Stress is another example. People react to stress with a wide range of outcomes. Sometimes people in the same family experience the same stresses but respond with different behaviours.

Stress can be described as symptoms of dysfunction that result from a person being unable to adapt to the varying challenges of the environment they live in. The body's energies (PEMS[2]) unbalance and the symptoms are a signal that the body has been unable to adapt. Left too long, other more serious problems may develop.

These patients are helped by medications and/or by chiropractic, osteopathic, physiotherapy, acupuncture, homeopathic, naturopathic or massage treatments. Different patients, according to their body types and beliefs, respond to the different or varying treatment regimes.

As practitioners, we often see people who at the end of many years of dysfunction have ended up in a position where life-prolonging treatments such as chemotherapy, radiotherapy or surgery are the last tools available to them.

Observations left me wondering why:

- People who were sick all their lives often lived for a long time
- People who ate well and who appeared healthy, fit, and happy often died early
- Mortality and sickness of health practitioners and health workers followed the same trends as the general public.

As a health professional, I wanted my patients to improve in health, and heal the way I understood the body should work. Naturally, hereditary family

---

2   *'PEMS' refers to the Physical, Emotional, Mental, and Spiritual energies.*

weaknesses and strengths had to be taken into consideration; however, I observed that stress appeared to be the common denominator that surfaced the experience of symptoms and ill health.

My conclusion was that there was more research needed to understand how the body worked and why it reacted differently for each person to the various challenges and stresses of our lives.

Various treatments – medication, herbs, nutrition, spinal and cranial adjustments, acupuncture, physical therapy and massage – aim to relieve symptoms, which satisfies the practitioner and the patient. But has the patient moved on to a better health pattern and has the body been able to heal and address the issues that caused the initial trouble?

Patients are changing the face of health care. In some countries, up to 50% of patients are seeking alternative therapies. Many people are challenging their doctors by being able to Google their diagnosis and condition. This can make doctors feel defensive or inadequate because along with the possibility of misinformation from the internet there is also no way that doctors can keep up with all the knowledge and advances in every condition.

Initially I followed the theory that the body heals itself providing you follow good basic health principles like eating good food, getting regular exercise, sleeping well, having healthy personal and family relationships, practising good personal hygiene and principles, and minimising stress.

I am not anti the allopathic (medical profession) approach. The advances in medicine and surgery are truly amazing and if it were not for such advances we would not have the quantity or quality of life we have grown to expect.

What is more important: quality or quantity of life?

There are many therapies out there, especially in the natural health range. These therapies appear to be best suited to functional problems of health. Allopathic, mainstream medicine is best suited to crisis and emergency (life/death) situations.

Functional health problems are not life-threatening. They are more chronic problems that the patient has experienced for years that have the potential to lead to more serious conditions. One can liken it to a car not starting properly, not idling, and just chugging along – if you don't get it fixed it may turn into a crisis/emergency situation. Crisis or emergency care is just that – emergency care to save life and limb. To use the car analogy – the car has broken down and won't go and so major intervention or new parts are needed.

There are four important factors in practitioner-patient relationships that can influence treatment and outcomes for both parties.

1. **Placebo** *(The Merck Manual, Eighteenth Edition, 2006):* A placebo is an inactive substance or treatment that is used in controlled studies for comparison with presumably active medication or treatment. Placebos are allegedly harmless and inert but may have profound effects, both positive and negative. Anticipation of results, suggestibility, faith or hope can account for up to 50% of symptom relief, or relief in 50% of patients.

2. **Intentionality:** Another form of placebo relates to the practitioner's expectation, belief, and faith in their treatment or medicines. This can account for up to another 50% of symptom relief. The doctor intends and expects the patient to respond to his/her therapy. Two different doctors can give the same medication with varying outcomes.

3. **Charisma:** Different patients respond to different doctor personalities. Characteristics that affect results include being caring, charming, understanding, considerate, and empathetic or equally include seeming uninterested, dismissive, entitled, arrogant, and rude.

4. **Therapy and Practice Identity:** Patients are drawn to different forms of therapy according to the type of treatment they identify with at that particular time; this can be due to current trends, social influences or other reasons, i.e. at some stage of their lives they may relate to a practitioner who prescribes pharmaceuticals or who specialises in nutrition or homeopathy and at another stage they may relate to someone who uses manual therapy, massage or counselling. Part of the treatment's success will be due to the person's current belief system.

Like all forms of healing, chiropractic adjustments and homeopathy have placebo effects and as a practitioner I do have intentionality with treatment regimes. It can be debated whether muscle testing is accurate as a single entity because of the intentionality of the tester – the practitioner wants to find answers. This does influence the outcome. Knowing this, I have endeavoured to be diligent in my testing. To further add significance, my intention has been to find patterns or trends that I can pass on to my associates for their use in treatment. Results and feedback from patients determine usefulness of new developments.

Once these patterns have been proven to be useful they are put into techniques. At times, it has been very challenging (almost to the point of exasperation) when trying to understand what the body is saying. The principle of, "what works is evidenced in results" has given me confidence, even if at this point in time we cannot accurately explain it in acceptable scientific terms.

"It's not that I'm so smart; it's just that I stay with problems longer."
(Albert Einstein)

Taking into consideration the above, I am always open to possibilities that expand to a broader base of understanding. The possibilities appear to be endless when studying humans.

The title 'human being' is interesting as it appears to be relevant as to who we are.

'Being' means an individual thing, a life, living, a soul, a spirit or an entity.

'Human' means mortal, manlike, fallible, imperfect, vulnerable, kind or natural.

We are a human body that is self-limiting and vulnerable, combined with an individual soul/spirit entity, which supposedly has purpose and immortality. This definition of human being helps us **understand more clearly who we are**.

CHAPTER 4

Early case histories

Three cases influenced my attitude and learning.

Jennifer's Case History

Jennifer, a forty-two-year-old woman, consulted me for chronic neck/back pain, headaches, digestive upsets, energy loss, plus frequent colds and flu. My testing showed farm chemical toxicity from 2,4-D, paraquat, lead, and arsenic.

Over several treatments, she responded well and asked if I would treat her three children aged nine, seven, and four years. The nine-year-old showed slight chemical toxicity, the seven-year-old had problems just like his Mum, and the four-year-old had no sign of toxicity. They were a farming family so I asked about chemicals. Jennifer's husband was a farmer but also a part-time agricultural spraying contractor. We now had the source of the problem, possibly from handling his work clothing. The children's symptoms and problems fitted exactly with the level of their respective toxicity.

A number of years later Jennifer, happy with her results, asked if I would see her husband who was having some back problems. I was interested to see him. His case-history form said that he had a sore back and neck following a car accident ten years prior. Questioning revealed he never got colds, flu, headaches, energy loss, rashes or any other symptoms that may relate to chemical toxicity. Testing showed some structural problems but I could not find anything that suggested any form of toxicity. He had been spraying chemicals for twenty-five years and in his own words was often "covered in it". I have seen many other similar cases that proved that chemical toxicity in patients does exist but I learned it was not the chemicals that were the problem; it was actually the way in which that person's body handled it. Twenty years later Jennifer's husband is still a farmer and other than occasional neck/back problems he functions well.

I'm not saying that chemical toxicity is not a problem in society generally, but it affects people differently, according to their make-up and constitution. Generally speaking, **if people are sensitive emotionally and mentally they will be sensitive physically.** This can perpetuate a 'Catch 22' situation as when they are physically unwell the mind becomes even more involved.

In this family, the father and two daughters were not as susceptible as the mother and son to the effects of chemicals in their bodies. Mother and son are very sensitive/knowing individuals.

Annabelle's Case History

A sixteen-year-old high school student, Annabelle consulted me for acute headaches, neck stiffness, recurring throat infections, abdominal discomfort, and dizziness/vertigo attacks. Through blood tests she had been diagnosed with glandular fever and had been unable to attend school for eight weeks; she spent most of her time in bed, too exhausted to do anything. Testing showed some metal toxicity due to nickel, silver, and mercury – confirmed by skin reactions around piercings in her ears. She also tested positive to the Epstein-Barr virus nosode[1] (the most common cause of glandular fever). Testing of her neck and spine showed muscular tightness but did not indicate that spinal manual therapy would be helpful.

Treatment consisted of my protocol in homeopathy for the metal and virus issues. Within two days she was feeling a lot better and was able to spend half the day out of bed – everyone was encouraged. On her next visit a similar treatment was administered but with little to no improvement – in fact the sore throat returned and she was relapsing.

---

1   Nosodes are homeopathic formulas made up from diseased tissue, fungi, viruses, bacteria, parasites, and chemicals.

A full investigation of the patient and her mother included questions along the lines of: "When did this start? What was going on in your life at that time or just prior to the onset? Have you experienced sickness before this time?"

Annabelle's glandular fever symptoms started when she was studying for exams eight weeks before. Four weeks prior to that, her grandmother had died suddenly. Gran lived with Annabelle's family and looked after the children and household while both parents worked. Annabelle was the oldest child and had a very close relationship with her grandmother. Her sore throats developed on the day of the funeral and the glandular fever set in four weeks later.

At that time, I was experimenting with magnets, trying to find how energy was behaving in the body. Any energy imbalances detected would relate to emotional/mental points that I had found in the body. My work was in its infancy but I had located fear, grief, anger, subservience, and guilt here. Combining these, I then treated Annabelle four more times over the next month for emotional/mental balance plus Epstein-Barr virus. Halfway through the treatment period she was able to attend school again and after several more visits over the next six months she was healthy and to my knowledge has never had a recurrence.

This case opened up my approach and learning. No matter what the condition you must always reward and balance the emotional/mental/ spiritual aspects as well as the physical. The body identifies with locating and correcting faults only when **the cause** of the problem is located. In this case, the emotional trauma was the origin or source of her glandular fever. (The Epstein-Barr virus relates to fear issues.)

Pete's Case History

Pete, a forty-eight-year-old long-haul truck driver, consulted me for chronic lower back and thoracic pain. He needed frequent visits to chiropractors, osteopaths, and physiotherapists to keep him capable of working (with treatment every week to two weeks). The problem was, in his opinion, worsening, and was costing him a lot of money as well as threatening his ability to keep working.

On examination, I could not find any major structural problems other than *that his whole spine was somewhat unstable due to what I thought had been overly frequent spinal treatments. He was unhappy with my analysis as I was not going to manually adjust him without finding evidence that it was needed. My findings showed that he was majorly anxious and stressed. He was not pleased with my findings and recommendations.*

We struck a deal that I would treat him and if he responded well he could pay me later and if not – no payment was due. Three months later he came in again, paid his account for his initial treatment as agreed. He said he hadn't been treated by anyone since seeing me but he didn't want "any of that hocus-pocus stuff" again about what was going on in his head. This time he showed evidence of needing some structural work. He also showed as needing emotional/mental balancing but I didn't go there. He paid before leaving this time!

A week later Pete was back saying, "Your treatment didn't work!" We struck another deal of no payment if my treatment didn't work this time. This time treatment consisted of some structural work plus balancing of his PEMS[2]. A month later there was a case of beer on the doorstep of the office with the fee in cash tucked inside it!

Ten years later he was still working hard, driving, lifting, and bending. A lot of positive things had happened since in his personal life. He followed a six-monthly check-up regime mainly for, in his words, "keeping my head right".

Pete moved to another city and I have not seen him for many years. He is hopefully happily retired and enjoying life.

These three cases stimulated me to investigate the emotional/mental/spiritual connection with physical health. The more answers I got, the more questions I had. That formula has not changed to this present day. My journey of learning is the basis of the Hale Technique.

Through my investigations using muscle testing I had found:
- Many points and combinations of points on the body that responded to magnets, lasers, vibration, and red and white strobe lights. The muscle response was either positive or negative, i.e. there was a normal response

---

2 *'PEMS' refers to the Physical, Emotional, Mental, and Spiritual energies.*

or an abnormal response. If abnormal, I had a new point. This took many hours and days of frustrating work learning what the body was trying to tell me.

- Whether these points related to emotional, mental, spiritual or physical origins.
- Once having established the point as being emotional or mental, what each of these points related to by spelling the words out, using muscle testing, and then looking the words up in dictionaries and investigating the meaning.

CHAPTER 5

Clearer picture

Although patients were very happy with results, I could not explain how and why it all fitted together to improve their health. Then around seventeen years ago, I met a spiritual mentor called Maureen Rose.

Maureen not only helped me grow personally through challenging me, but also explained why what I had found worked. She gave me understanding by explaining behavioural patterns. Her insight was simply amazing, not only from her own colourful journey through life, which was very similar to mine, but also because she had a level of knowing that I have never encountered before or since.

We argued on almost every meeting but that is what a mentor is about. Counsellors hear your story and prompt your coming to a healthy conclusion. Mentors challenge you to change your beliefs, attitudes, and behaviours so that you alter your outcomes.

Maureen was a key figure as I put this technique together. I gradually came to understand that we are all unique individuals who think, feel, and know differently. When we become unbalanced the body knows how, and in what order, to restore balance for optimum health (via a unique recipe or coding). What I have found is a way to challenge the body to let the practitioner in, to find pathways that lead to the source of what help each person uniquely needs. Each treatment can be likened to an onion skin, peeling back layers, sometimes with a few tears! The development and pathways are an ongoing journey into knowledge, an open-ended experience in learning.

Maureen not only helped me understand human behaviour, but also explained how my findings fitted into each patient's health picture. Through her spiritual ability, she was able to explain how the mind, emotionally and mentally, was influencing each patient's well-being. Her insight was often very different to the patient's story. Testing with this insight led me to develop new techniques with effective treatment outcomes.

We shared many patients. She would challenge the patient on their beliefs and behaviour, which gave them the chance to accept and understand their problem. She could then give me the information about the patient's issues and was subsequently able to tell me what techniques I needed to develop to complement her challenge. At times, it seemed impossible, but somehow it came together. I was enlightened. The patient's health would improve and all three of us would be happy with the results.

An example of such a case could be a patient who may have thought that their Dad (who was abusive and had addiction issues) was the person they needed to deal with. However, with new knowledge, testing of the body showed that Mum was the person involved, due to abandonment and betrayal issues. As an adult, the patient saw Dad as the problem but when they were experiencing these issues they were a child. From a child's perspective, Mum can do and make everything right. The energy block came from those experiences when Mum let the patient down by not changing Dad and the consequences of his behaviour.

Maureen would tell me this from her knowledge and insight. I would have to find a pathway into the body to elicit this information. The patient was informed and had new understanding. My job was to find and balance the associated energy imbalances around this issue. Once corrected, we observed health improvements to issues that had plagued patients for years.

The healing is related to understanding and forgiving Mum as she was suffering too, not being able to protect herself and her children without adverse consequences. The Hale Technique treatment balances the energies of the four aspects of PEMS[1]; reinforcing a new beginning of past traumas and experiences.

---

1   'PEMS' refers to the Physical, Emotional, Mental, and Spiritual energies.

In Maureen's words, "I can find the underlying issues, but I cannot correct the energies to allow the patients to heal; that is why I send them to you." We worked together on hundreds of patients over a fifteen-year experience of enlightenment, learning, and experimentation.

Many problems were solved by balancing brain and/or hormonal chemistry with nutrition, or else referring them to their GP with a suggestion of a certain pre-tested effective antidepressant medication. At first, because of my beliefs and philosophies, I was very anti the use of antidepressant medication. However, when managed and maintained with treatment (to balance PEMS) I was and still am amazed at the changes in patients' lives and health.

After an eight-year battle with multiple cancers in her body, Maureen passed away aged forty-nine years in early 2015. Many of her friends and family agree that she gave away all her energies to her clients. This is a fault often observed in people who are spiritually gifted. She experienced a horrific childhood and adolescence, but through accepting help achieved an ultimate level of healing to help others. Unfortunately for herself she would never accept help from other people unless she was the one who was controlling the process – one of those other people was me. This became a source of debate between us over the years as she never let me into a level deeper than physical.

CHAPTER 6

Body-Mind balance

The Hale Technique is designed to address the patient's health through a body-mind balance approach. Not only does it treat the patient, but it also gives a pathway for healing.

Assessment of each patient is firstly by way of observation – how they walk, talk, and behave, plus listening to them, questioning them – in combination with a case history. Clinical tests lead to further evaluation. Muscle testing (Applied Kinesiology or AK), including intuition and intentionality from the practitioner should complete a picture of proposed treatment planning, and probable prognosis (predicted outcomes of treatment). Not all patients are taken on. Between three and six visits are proposed to those we can help, after which time further evaluation may be needed.

Muscle testing does have its faults – because of the intentions and charisma of the practitioner – however it should be used in conjunction with case history, examination, and clinical findings. It is not a cure-all, nor is it, in my opinion, a diagnostic tool – but rather another tool in the practitioner's toolbox. A modern-day carpenter will have all the latest battery-operated tools but he/she should still be able to use a hammer, chisel, handsaw, plane, etc. In most cases, however, muscle testing (AK) is better than guessing.

Often patients come in refusing to take medication because it is causing them some issues. It's helpful for the patient if we test their medication and nutritional products for effectiveness and possible side effects. Medication, while it is needed and helpful, may cause side effects for that particular patient. Testing the patient with exposure to that medication can display such side effects, which most often can be alleviated or neutralised by using complex homeopathy. We cannot prescribe or change medication, nor can we advise patients not to take it. However, if we can't neutralise it, we can have a conversation with the prescribing doctor where we can discuss the possibility of finding an alternative.

Neurotransmitter levels in the brain and nervous system are also very important for assessment, and occasionally medication is either neutralised or changed for this reason too. This has led to life-changing outcomes for patients.

The Hale Technique works in conjunction with other forms of healthcare. It is not a panacea but an adjunct, which because of its ability to communicate enhances all treatments. Symptom relief can be achieved temporarily by balancing energy, but personal growth and healing require the patient's ownership and acceptance of themselves, their world, and their behaviour.

CHAPTER 7

Key influences

S everal people and techniques have been influential in the development of the Hale Technique.

Applied Kinesiology (AK)

Applied Kinesiology was my introduction to muscle testing in the early 1970s. Founded by chiropractor Dr George Goodheart Jr in 1964, Applied Kinesiology is used by many practitioners as a diagnosis and treatment format. However, I think of it more as a tool to help with assessment. Nevertheless, Applied Kinesiology is the most important tool in the kit of the Hale Technique. It allows assessment, diagnosis, and more importantly a personalised treatment plan for the practitioner, in the sequence of patient healing, as the practitioner can ask the body what to treat next, in order of priority.

Something George was often heard to quote was:

> *"If the only tool you have is a hammer,*
> *then every problem looks like a nail."*
> *(Abraham Maslow)*

(If your ability to learn, to be open to change, and to gain new skills and knowledge is limited then what you have to offer, to others, will be limited to the same degree.)

Sacro Occipital Technique (SOT)

SOT was developed by Major Bertrand DeJarnette, a chiropractor, in the 1920s. It incorporates non-force osteopathic and chiropractic principles/ techniques to correct spinal dysfunction by restoring synchronised movement between the skull (cranium), pelvis (sacrum iliums and coccyx), and spine. A popular technique has evolved from these techniques and principles called Cranio-Sacral Therapy.

Neuro Emotional Technique (NET)

Chiropractor Dr Scott Walker founded NET in the late 1980s. It addresses physical and behavioural stress-related conditions that relate to past physical/ psychological trauma. NET is based on the physiological foundation of stress-related responses that are recorded in the body at a physical level, and which display as acute/chronic symptoms.

Dr Sheldon Deal

A chiropractor and naturopath, Sheldon was one of the founders/teachers of Applied Kinesiology and 'Touch for Health' as a system of analysis and treatment. He introduced advanced levels of nutrition and various energy tools (such as magnets and lasers) into treatment protocol. These tools facilitated shortcuts in Applied Kinesiology protocol. Sheldon's idea to use various energy tools opened up for me new horizons of communication, challenges to the body, and understanding. Sheldon is a great teacher, practitioner, lateral thinker, innovator, and communicator.

Dr John O'Malley

John worked as an associate at Integrated Health for eight years. During that time, he gained his PhD in Chiropractic Philosophy. We had many interesting discussions and conversations on philosophy and chiropractic. We saw eye-to-eye on most topics. He spoke from an educated viewpoint; I spoke from intuitive knowledge and yet we both agreed, usually arriving at the same conclusion. John gave me further understanding of 'intentionality' (O'Malley, 1998) and how it plays a major part in treatment and so results in patient care. (See 'Intentionality'.)

Robin Woodsford

Robin is a 'Breathwork Psychotherapist' who I first consulted in the late 80s. He has become a great friend through our mutual association as practitioner/patient. Being the only male therapist I had ever been touched by, he exposed my childhood abuse issues and helped me revisit and own those experiences. There were some tough times but Robin paved the way. He is a master of his profession and is truly passionate about people and their lives, his work, his learning, and life as an expression of love and self-fulfilment.

I loved the sign on the back of his door (a widely-used pun in psychology):

Denial is not a river in Egypt.
(Unknown)

Brian O'Hagan

Brian was a practical, inspirational, and multi-talented born leader who could turn his talents from being a healer, adviser, counsellor, to then handling large engineering projects. His last years were spent as a senior instructor in fixed-wing aircraft and helicopters.

He successfully led the Government's 'Commission of inquiry into Chiropractic Report, 1979' as President of the New Zealand Chiropractic Association, which became a milestone in acceptance of chiropractic treatment worldwide.

We in the chiropractic profession all admire Brian and thank him for his efforts, and success in his many achievements, not only as a chiropractor but also as a talented leader. Finding the time and energy to do all he did along with being a husband and a Dad must have been challenging.

His efforts changed many people's lives – one of those lucky people was me. Thank you, Brian.

Maureen Rose

Maureen Rose was my great mentor. She challenged me to see the people who abused me as a child as my teachers. As she would say, "You chose them and look what you have achieved in life and how you are able to help and understand others now. Instead of wallowing in self-pity you need to thank them." (See 'Spiritual Side'.) Initially I really struggled with this challenge.

Learning to think this way didn't heal me immediately, but it did change my life. She would say, "You have done over twenty years counselling, etc. While you can *accept* and *acknowledge* the past, how are you going to *heal* unless you understand and forgive your perpetrators?"

Later Maureen proved to be extremely helpful in my work with patients; she would give me great insight into my experimentation. My findings would say one thing but Maureen would tell me that they meant something else and upon rechecking I'd find that the body would indeed agree with Maureen's analysis. This way I learned how my beliefs, through *intentionality*, initially would show only what I knew and therefore wanted to find – confined by the boundaries of my knowledge and experience at that time.

An example of such a case might be that initially I would find anxiety, persecution, and abandonment in the patient, which all related to their family members. This trend would continue to occur again and again. Maureen would then see the patient and advise me that the issue was repeating because the real issue was subservience (be reasonable; do it my way), anxiety, and righteousness (jealousy-related). The patient was controlling and bossy and so the family reacted by withdrawing and becoming rebellious. My initial findings supported the patient's victimhood. When I was made aware, I could treat the energies supporting what Maureen had found, which were the energies that needed balancing before the patient could move forward. The patient was challenged, the energies balanced, giving the patient the opportunity to understand, heal through changing their behaviour, and eventually forgive.

Over time, I learned to accept these challenges and eventually we could talk the same language; during the latter years, we never had any confrontations. What a teacher! Certainly not for the light-hearted – as all who knew her came to appreciate.

CHAPTER 8

How the Hale Technique works

What is the Hale Technique?

The Hale Technique has developed over the last thirty years through observing the body, challenging it, and trying to understand how it works.

Applied Kinesiology (muscle testing) has been a major contributor in the formation of a language we can use to communicate with the body.

As a practitioner, I didn't want to rely solely on the usual pattern of patient symptom presentation followed by clinical tests and physical examination as I knew that this pattern often did not lead to an accurate diagnosis with a possible treatment plan. My muscle testing results challenged me majorly as:

- My beliefs systems were not very adaptable, especially when the body indicated that the source of the problem was the mind, rather than the physical body – with all its chemistry and all its anatomical and structural possibilities.
- When communicating with the body using muscle testing, yes or no are the only answers.

The first challenge has been to not only ask the right questions, but also to come up with the vast array of possible answers. The second challenge is accepting and understanding that that is the answer. The next challenge is how to develop a technique to address that energy.

Once I had developed a technique, that technique was then taught to my associate practitioners. Subsequently, from feedback on the results observed, we were able to establish the worth of each technique. Over the years only 20% of these techniques have been retained and used. As I grow and develop newer techniques, a lot of the old ones are superseded.

How does it work?

Almost every potential patient who consults our office presents with an over-active mental mind.

The amount of energy in the body is a constant at any one time. This energy is distributed throughout the four main areas of the body (PEMS[1]) in varying amounts. Therefore, if there is a high in one area there has to be corresponding lows in the other three areas. The mental mind is the most powerful and so it usually wins the battle, unless there is a crisis in the physical, emotional, or spiritual energies. In this case, they take precedence over the mental energy.

Examples of crises in the physical, emotional or spiritual energies are: heightened physical activity, emotional excitement, survival or competitive situations, etc.

Normally the patient does not have to tell the practitioner what is happening for them, although this is helpful. Through measuring the levels of PEMS, the practitioner can further determine the levels of anxiety, depression, melancholy, hormones, neurotransmitters, toxicity in the body, etc.

From this, the practitioner can now ask the body what technique is best to restore and balance the four systems to equal amounts of energy. The practitioner can now tell the patient what technique appears most suitable. The patient usually exclaims, "How do you know that?" The practitioner's answer is, "Your body said that is what is going on for you."

The symptoms and experience should fit the technique chosen by the practitioner. These techniques are multiple. Some examples of the issues needing treatment techniques are: various types of anxiety, issues with personal identity, nervous breakdown, hopelessness, feeling overwhelmed, need for nurture, forgiveness, grief, hostility, being frightened/terrified, control issues or any of the emotional issues listed further on in the book.

---

1   'PEMS' refers to the Physical, Emotional, Mental, and Spiritual energies.

The technique is better explained to the patient at the completion of treatment as a full picture cannot be gained until the practitioner has all the related information. The spiritual energy provides **who and what** the technique related to; the emotional/mental energy gives information about **feelings, choices, and experience**; the physical energy should relate to **symptoms experienced by the body** with regards to function, pain, discomfort, and loss of function, hormonal or immune systems faults.

Sometimes patients get stuck in their beliefs and refuse to move out of their mental controlling way of being. In these cases, we may suggest various forms of counselling, psychotherapy, completion letters, plus other 'in house' techniques that help them communicate, maybe for the first time in their life. Balancing their PEMS energies only gives temporary relief if they do not take ownership of their behaviour and issues. As practitioners, we help your body heal physical, emotional, and spiritual energies but we cannot *change* how you think (mental). We can only *challenge* that energy.

If the patient is stuck the treatment still works as the energy has been balanced but because the patient isn't willing to change, we observe the same problem or similar problems emerging again and again. Some patients prefer to stay stuck, saying, "The treatment is the only relief that I get for my symptoms!" Sometimes these patients decide to move on in life, but often they just move to another treatment source as the years go by.

"You are the only common denominator in your problem. You pay for my time and advice – not the results. I am here to help. It is up to you as you have the problem – not me!"
(Bryan Hale)

The secret of treatment lies in the emotional/spiritual energy balancing as it gives the practitioner and patient information as to who and what the treatment relates to. An added advantage is that it gives the practitioner ammunition that may be needed to challenge the patient 'face-to-face' with what *the body is saying* is the issue ... and not what the patient *thinks* is the issue.

"You can think what you want
but you can't always feel what you want."
(Bryan Hale)

As practitioners, we can only challenge your body and ask what it is saying. With treatment, the patient has the opportunity to change and to move to a better level of health and learning.

Synopsis

The biggest help in healing is to own your own behaviour.

Formula: accepting, understanding, and owning how you behave is the key to improving your overall health, happiness, success, self-worth, relationships, and communications.

If someone else is able to point out aspects of your behavioural trait, i.e. trust, jealousy/righteousness, controlling, martyrdom, approval, anger, subservience, anxiety, fear, sadness, etc., *then by listening, accepting, and understanding* **that is how others perceive your behaviour,** *ownership* **becomes the first but also the biggest step in changing that behaviour (providing you want to).**

Your behaviour changes just by acknowledging and owning the facts.

People will read this and hopefully learn to change their world and surroundings, by solely looking at themselves. The more likely scenario is that they will use this information to diagnose other people's issues! This is good too as it leads to tolerance and understanding of others, which eventually may lead to challenging loved ones to acknowledge their behaviour, how it affects their health, and also how it affects the lives of those who are trying to love and support them.

CHAPTER 9

Treatment protocol

Prospective patients often ask, "What does the treatment involve?" when treated with the Hale Technique.

A précis of treatment is as follows:

- Following case history, initial examination, tests, and evaluation of the patient, the practitioner can now start asking questions of the body in relation to the varying energies, organ function and production, nervous system, immune system, hormone and neurotransmitter levels, etc. A lot of information can be gained through questioning the body with muscle testing, using language the body identifies with. This information needs to be correlated with the patient's presenting complaints and symptoms. Over the years, I have developed many techniques to stop the body from leading the practitioner down the wrong road. The body's protective instincts are understandable as it has been adapting and coping for years – in an attempt to keep everything functioning to its potential – in response to all the varying stresses encountered in life thus far.

- Usually on the first treatment, the body will not let the practitioner in very far (usually only at a physical level), however on subsequent treatments the body is very keen to display, in order of priority, the faults within.

- Once the practitioner has permission from the patient's body to assess and enter its energy fields, muscle testing is used to choose the appropriate technique that the body is displaying as needing. Once the technique is introduced, a temporary blockage of all energies in the body is observed by the practitioner, which confirms that the right technique has been chosen. The blockage is now neutralised with complex homoeopathy developed by myself.

- Following this procedure, the spiritual system now shows what the technique displays in relation to specific persons (Mum, Dad, partner, siblings, in-laws, etc.), place (where it happened), or things (circumstances, etc.) relating to the event.

- Now the physical system opens up to be treated. The patient is checked for the possibility of inflammation, infection, immune system faults, allergy-type reactions, and hormonal imbalances. In the case of involvement in the three 'i's' above, homeopathic nosodes[1] are used to treat the problem (this is helpful as the symptoms and the nosodes should match, e.g. Epstein-Barr virus – tiredness, bowel nosodes for digestive issues, pneumonia nosodes for respiratory conditions, etc.). Allergic substances such as antigens, pollens, etc. are tested on the body and if applicable are neutralised with complex homeopathy. Similarly, most major hormones relating to thyroid, adrenal glands, liver, pancreas, ovaries, and testes are tested and neutralised as above.

- After completing the physical balance, the emotional system displays first, followed by a mirror image by the mental system, both needing energy balancing. This aspect of treatment is very helpful as over two to three treatments it displays various emotional/mental faults that keep repeating. Along with the spiritual display, the practitioner now gets a picture of not only the emotional/mental fault, but also of who these faults relate to. This is our opportunity to challenge the patient on their repetitive behavioural traits. Sometimes it is not easy for the patient to move on, but it explains why the faults and health issues repeat. Many times, it helps (via clarification by the spiritual system), who and what these issues relate to. Patients often want to argue, but the body has a different slant. The problem is not going to get better while the patient holds on to the same old story. It is important to look at it differently – from the angle the body

---

1   *Nosodes are homeopathic formulas made up from diseased tissue, fungi, viruses, bacteria, parasites, and chemicals.*

has interpreted rather than from the story the mental mind has made up to fit in with a pattern of continued victimhood. Once a mindset change is accepted and eventually understood by the patient, healing can now begin.

(Like the earlier example where a patient may have blamed their father for thirty years as the cause of their victimhood. The reality, according to the body is that the issue is actually with their Mum. It never got better as they were looking at the wrong picture. When you deal with the you-Mum relationship all the energies start to open up and heal.) **At the end of the day, it all boils down to your issues with yourself and your world – family and surroundings are just the teaching energies you chose to learn and experience from in this lifetime.**

- Now the spiritual system again shows as it did in the first instance.
- The practitioner can now ask the body if all that needed to be done has been done. If the body affirms this, there is a procedure for exiting the body, detoxing on the way out and apologising for changing the energies! (Interestingly, this is the same procedure used if a patient has reacted or not recovered well after an anaesthetic/operation.)
- Through experience we have learned that the practitioner has to actively look for any structural faults in the cranium (skull), pelvis or spine. These faults need to be corrected before the patient leaves the office as we have found that the patient often experienced chronic, sometimes acute pain within hours of leaving the office if those faults were not corrected at the time of treatment for PEMS[2] balancing. Almost every patient needs a structural correction following treatment, which may not only include the above-mentioned areas but also may include the TMJ (jaw), shoulders, feet, iliolumbar ligament syndrome, dropped kidney syndrome, and diaphragm imbalances. Following these corrections, the spiritual system shows it needs to be balanced again in accordance with the previous criteria found throughout previous energy balancing/treatment. This demonstrates how the structure reflects the energy imbalances throughout the body, illustrating why people experience pain relief, increased mobility, improved function of all body systems – when treated physically to relieve suppressed

2 *'PEMS' refers to the Physical, Emotional, Mental, and Spiritual energies.*

energy and expression with spinal, cranial, and pelvic adjustments, performed by chiropractors, osteopaths, and more recently some physiotherapists. This type of treatment releases and changes energies, sometimes enough that it produces wonderful results just by performing treatment(s) solely. In chronic, more complex health situations there is more input needed to balance those energies.

- If a patient presents with an acute structural problem of the neck, back, pelvis, shoulder, etc. the body requests the aforementioned PEMS[3] balancing (set out above) be completed before any structural work is attempted. We can treat just structurally, but it requires multiple visits and time (as opposed to just one or two visits) to clear up long-term structural problems.

- At this time, the patient is checked for the possible need to take nutritional supplementation in support of tissue, organ, hormonal, and emotional/mental deficiencies. We also check medications and nutritional supplements for the possible need to neutralise side-effects.

In addition, foods intolerance, malabsorption, and reactions are checked. Total elimination of gluten is a major issue for those who are affected, as it causes inflammation in the body generally. The worst effect is on the brain and nervous system, secondly the digestive system. I agree that it is sometimes over-diagnosed but for those affected great changes are observed when they **totally eliminate** any gluten-containing products. These days it is not as difficult to comply with.

Dairy intolerance is not common but is more difficult to stay away from as many foods contain traces of dairy. Dairy malabsorption is easier as various forms of lactase (enzyme that breaks down lactose) are available commercially. Babies and young children are often sensitive to eggs and many other products. In adults, children, and babies we observe (with treatment over a period of a few years) their food intolerances, other than gluten and lactose, disappear. I have experimented with anaphylactic food reactions but at this point in time there is nothing I can add. Crisis-care kits are an essential for these people to carry everywhere with them.

---

3   'PEMS' refers to the Physical, Emotional, Mental, and Spiritual energies.

- The patient is then advised on a time frame for their next treatment/ treatments. Most cases require four to six treatments before starting maintenance treatment. Maintenance care can be anywhere between one month to six months (usually two, three or four months).

  Maintenance treatment is the secret to staying well and continuing to grow as a person, improving one's general health and well-being. Most patients request to come back sooner than the recommended three- to four-month interval suggested by their practitioner as they say, "I can't seem to last that long, and I am not about to go backwards now that I have come this far."

- We practitioners are usually checked weekly when in working mode as the treatment is emotionally draining and very taxing at times. As a team, we also need debriefing, plus I appreciate trying out my new techniques on my associates, which leads to informative feedback!!

- I am a very proud chiropractor and I very much value the healing power of chiropractic treatment. I have always taken a step further than most as I have an unceasing desire to learn and understand more about how the body works and wants to heal.

CHAPTER 10

Beliefs

A belief is an idea which is true for you in your personal experience. There are three components to forming a belief:

1. **Upbringing:** You are exposed to ideas, beliefs, and prejudices from family, friends, and schooling. You witness how elders and peers use these to gain or lose power in their lives.
2. **Life experience:** You form opinions on how you deal with life and also on how you want to be perceived. Your own belief system is a contract between your mental and emotional minds. This can either challenge or confirm what you were taught by your family.

> *"Therefore, a belief is a contract between what you think and how you feel about that thought. If it feels right, fits into your experiences, and holds some purpose, you develop a belief."*
> *(Bryan Hale)*

3. **Mental influence:** Once the belief forms you can use it to your advantage or disadvantage by:
   Improving self-worth by belonging to a group, aligning to like-minded individuals, or by creating focus and purpose in your life through goals, aims, and objectives. This focus can be powerful enough to achieve what was thought impossible (in sport, business, personal, leadership, etc. matters).

Or

In the negative, you can choose to be righteous by being critical of how and what others believe, therefore judging them and persecuting them for believing something different.

A belief is neither right nor wrong, good nor bad; nor is it finite. Issues come when beliefs give rise to righteousness, persecution, martyrdom, abuse or addiction.

For healthier outcomes, we need healthier desires and beliefs. These are often the result of education, through which we develop empathy, under-standing, tolerance, and acceptance. Education offers a stronger and more positive approach to life, resulting in us choosing freedom/happiness and allowing others to do the same.

A belief is a choice that can be changed. If you are willing to accept life's lessons and use them to change, your thinking will eventually alter your belief system. For example, you may believe that the opposite sex can never be trusted. Then you meet someone of the opposite sex who is very nice and this relationship shows they can be trusted. Your belief is then challenged and you now have a choice to change your belief or stay locked in fear. Many stay, feeling that it is easier to go with the flow, than to take the risk and stand up and be true to their values and principles. This is a symptom of 'fear of success'.

Conscious choice is one of the greatest assets of the mind. If you come to the end of your life with the same set of beliefs you inherited from your family, you may feel cheated that you did not live or experience your own life to its fullest potential.

CHAPTER 11

Instincts

B asic instincts relate closely to the five basic senses. Smell to love, touch to power, sight to freedom, hearing to survival, taste to fun. The five main instincts are: survival, love, power, freedom, and fun.

Instincts are natural, intuitive, inborn responses that form our unique personality as a human being. Basic instincts are evident in all of us but the differences come from the strengths and weaknesses of our individual responses. Instincts are carried by the spiritual system, but the spiritual system can't express itself as an entity so therefore we transfer that spiritual energy into emotional energy. This way instincts can be integrated into the mind to keep us safe, as well as free to experience love, to learn, and to have fun.

"Instincts are genetically hardwired behaviours that enhance
our ability to cope with vital environmental experiences."
(Bryan Hale)
(For example, fear of snakes, spiders, insects, etc.)

Instincts also connect to our physical body through programming and development in utero. This way they become genetically coded into the DNA of organs and the nervous system (brain, spinal cord, and nerves). Using survival as an example, we breathe and protect ourselves in times of crisis without thinking or analysing. It is instinctive in our body.

With the instincts connecting through emotions, the mental mind can now get involved too. Mentally we have the ability to act out basic instinctive responses, or to create negative outcomes from choices. When we are focused on using them at a physical, emotional, and spiritual level we express ourselves in a productive way. However, because of the choices involved in using the mental mind we can develop self-destruction from survival, depression from love, victimhood from power, martyrdom from freedom, and sadness from fun; these are frequent expressions of behaviour when we are bored, complacent, or too comfortable in our lives.

> *"Survival is supposedly our strongest instinct.*
> *However, observation shows self-destruction*
> *is often stronger. We all eventually die."*
> *(Bryan Hale)*

CHAPTER 12

Values

*"A value is a principle – an ideal or a philosophy
that has personal significance and meaning."*
(Bryan Hale)

Every individual has a core set of personal values, which come from one's spirituality. These values help form one's beliefs, one's boundaries, one's personalities, one's character, and also one's self-worth.

*"There are many different ways to raise your children;
but as long as you prioritise teaching them to be
accountable, gracious, and have good values
they will become good citizens."*
(Maureen Rose)

Values come from the deepest level of existence and are therefore more powerful than opinions and attitudes. Without values, we would be animal-like, living our lives by following our urges, whims, and passions. We would have very little regard for ourselves or others and be devoid of the truths we hold dear. Our values are the origin of what make us human beings, the superior primate on planet Earth.

Some of the more common values are:

Accountability, ambition, cleanliness, commitment, communication, compassion, competition, concern for others, courage, delight, dignity, discipline, empathy, equality, excellence, fairness, faithfulness, family, freedom, friendship, fun, goodness, gratitude, hard work, harmony, honesty, honour, hope, independence, individuality, integrity, leadership, learning, loyalty, not judging, openness, orderliness, personal growth, progress and improvement, prosperity, punctuality, respect, responsibility, results oriented, service to others, simplicity, success, sympathy, tolerance, trust, truth, and unity.

Values are expressions of our spiritual, personalised truths that fulfil us in what we do, how we see ourselves, and how we see others see us; as an individual, or as part of a group in our greater worldly influence and participation.

It can be difficult to live according to values because most people have never looked at themselves at this level. As humans, we tend to believe and act with a pack mentality, going with the flow because it is easier and doesn't require too much energy, input or conflict. We can still be an individual within the pack and through one's values influence the way the group acts and reacts. This way we activate others' consciousness, bringing their values to the surface to effect change.

Values govern the principle of, "Do unto others as you would have them do to you".

CHAPTER 13

Emotions

E motions are heartfelt, i.e. they essentially come from the heart and we can express any emotion by saying, "I feel".

"The best and most beautiful things in the world cannot be seen or even touched. They must be felt with the heart."
(Helen Keller)

There are varying levels and depths of emotions accordingly in all mammals. Humans act and react chiefly on emotions until our analytical mind (mental mind) develops somewhere between four to six years old. Until this time, we observe a wide range of behaviours according to that child's level of emotionality. We rarely see a child over the age of six years throwing a tantrum in public as they can be negotiated with in a logical (mental) fashion – avoiding a confrontational situation for all present.

Humans have two components of the mind:
1. The emotional (the subconscious)
2. The mental (the conscious)

Generally speaking, all other mammals have only an emotional side. This is why animals are unpredictable to the untrained handler as they do not possess an analytical (mental) mind and therefore cannot be reasoned or negotiated with. They can be trained to reproduce certain behaviours for rewards usually – food and love. Observation also shows that animals do not feel guilt as we humans do. This lack of guilt does exist in humans with certain personality disorders, e.g. psychopaths; they show little to no remorse for their murderous deeds.

The subconscious part of your mind is emotionally based and although it is continuously working throughout the twenty-four hours of the day, it is more apparent when the mental mind is less dominant, i.e. when we are at rest, at sleep, under the influence of alcohol or drugs or temporarily emotionally aroused (high-excitement situations). The intent of an emotion is basically positive, but the interplay with the mental mind can turn that into a negative intent. The mental mind gives us the choice as to how we express our emotional state at the time. For example:

- Experience of death to a small child is intriguing and fascinating, usually without emotional expression, whereas to an older child or adolescent there is meaning through association in their life.
- Humour is initiated by an unexpected ending or result. We usually have to explain to a young child why everyone is laughing. Once they learn about the situation they experience the humour too. Children love jokes, especially if *they* tell them. This is a way of being accepted and protected in 'the pack'.

Essentially, emotions are:
- Non-analytical
- Protection moderators
- A connection to spiritual side
- Something that gives us sympathy/empathy/compassion (most often from experiencing them)
- Heartfelt
- Relate to self-worth
- A display of basic instincts
- A result of an accumulation of series of events and situations that give meaning
- Easily altered to fit in with the mental and physical aspects of the body.

Non-Analytical – We don't analyse emotionally. We just feel, and nothing can change that feeling until the mental mind or instincts kick in to change how we see the situation. Emotions are very adaptable if challenged.

Protectors/Moderators – Often we think something, but our emotional state will bring in values and standards that challenge us or make us look at our motives or intents. This aspect looks at treating others how we would like others to treat us. Security and safety issues are self-protective; ultimately it is all about ME.

Connection to Spiritual Side – Means by which the spiritual side can be expressed through feelings and mind control. One's personality becomes evident in the way we express our emotions, in caring for oneself, and for those close to you.

Give us sympathy, empathy, and compassion – Sympathy is a natural emotive response for most, however empathy goes a step further as to have empathy you have to have experienced the same or a similar experience yourself. This creates a deeper level of emotion since because of our history and experiences we have felt the same pain of that particular feeling, e.g. death of a loved one. Compassion is even deeper and through experience and knowledge you live and teach this spiritual (Soul) lesson to others.

Heartfelt – Emotions only relate to you. You may feel for others but it is only a reflection of your feelings for yourself. For example:

a) You 'think' you are angry with someone else but you are only angry at yourself because you can't control that person.

b) You are at a funeral for your friend's parent. Your grief is for yourself in reflection of you losing one of your parents or you personally dying. The feeling and demonstration of grief is for yourself.

Self-worth relates back to your spirituality. However, to give self-worth meaning in your body you have to first **feel** you are worthy before you can **think** you are worthy. This gives it tangible meaning towards forming a belief that you are actually worthy, i.e. if you come into this world with low self-esteem and self-worth, it is very difficult to attain the emotional/mental level. This may be one of life's challenges when trying to achieve purpose of fulfilment (true purpose) in life.

Display of Basic Instincts – Comes through our emotions and spirituality to create autonomic (nervous system) reflexes and reactions, e.g. fight or flight, nurture, reality, etc. Examples are feelings of nausea, headaches, anxiety, and stress.

Accumulation of series of events and situations that give meaning – Often a parent comes up in treatment relating to 'forgiveness issues'. The parent may have died thirty years ago, but the patient's eyes fill with tears. They exclaim that they have dealt with this issue. The body says "yes", that they have dealt with it **mentally**, but not **emotionally**, **physically** or **spiritually** – therefore this energy has to be balanced. This may apply to an ex-husband/wife/partner or brother/sister. With balancing such energies in treatment, major symptoms like chronic back/neck pain, migraine, digestive upsets, etc. substantially decrease or disappear. The emotional system has locked in those feelings that relate to 'self-forgiveness', not so much forgiveness of others. (See 'Forgiveness'.)

Easily altered to fit in with the mental and physical aspects of the body – When you reverse the situation and imagine yourself as the perpetrator and the other person as the victim then you may see or appreciate a different story or picture, taking into consideration their experiences, their knowledge, their situation, and their intent. This can change your feeling about how you interpret the said situation (understanding). This is typical when patients are dealing with their parents' behaviour and treatment when they were growing up. Isn't it ironic that we begin to understand our parents once we have children of our own? Maybe they were just doing their very best with the knowledge, experience, and resources they had at that time and situation.

Emotions relate only to ourselves personally. Everything revolves around us. Because of our mental mind and conditioning, we don't want others to see us in a bad light. Our thinking and reasoning will always give us a story that protects our pride and self-esteem. When we test the body (without the mental mind involved) it disagrees by saying, "It is all about me totally, in every way, shape, and form. Consideration and giving to others is good, as long as it serves me well."

There appears to be only four basic emotions that we act or react to positively or negatively. There are many more emotions that we can name, but the ones set out in this book are the ones I have found to be most relevant to the healing formulas presented.

Trust is also a major emotion, but it is what I call a 'blanket emotion' as it is often an accompanying issue involved in most emotional/mental mind experiences.

Most human emotions emanate from the four listed below.
- Love
- Anger
- Jealousy
- Fear

Love

Love is the most talked about emotion, but also probably the most misunderstood emotion. Love can conquer any negative emotional situation. We crave love from others but also for ourselves, as without self-love we cannot give love to others nor can we receive love from others. In my experience, we need to do some form of 'personal development' or 'learning' in order to realise that self-love is the key to being able to give or receive love. Volumes of information have been published on this topic. Listed below are some explanations of what we see as practitioners, that may help clarify how love presents in our life.

Most people perceive love as being positive, caring, passionate, and also the building block of strong relationships. However, love can also be negative as seen in behaviour that leads to killing or controlling others, creating anxiety and depression, following addiction patterns, committing crimes of passion, destroying relationships both personally and in families, just to mention a few. As previously mentioned, emotions are all about you personally. "If I can't have you for myself, no one else is going to have you." (How often have we read or heard that as a reason for family violence?) "I will get your attention and love even if I have to make myself sick and depressed." "As I have missed out on your love, I now transfer my love to my behaviour of hiding myself away in my addictive ways so that now I love my alcohol, drugs, gambling, sex, etc. more than I love you and myself." Importantly, self-love is missing, usually because of a person's mental story or choice to live out of reality and become a victim.

A common issue we see relating to love is: **Ransom**.

This aspect of love comes about when a love connection ends due to death, sickness, the end of a relationship, etc.

Mentally the patient would deny that God[1] or someone owes them a ransom for the love they have lost, however the other aspects of the body disagree as: "Someone is going to have to pay me back for my lost love; it is not fair and so justice must be done." This aspect of love relates very strongly to grief, hopelessness, anger, fear, approval, trust, etc. When people understand this aspect of love it is easy to own our behaviour even though the mental mind disagrees. Ownership eventually leads to forgiveness. We often observe anger/resentment in conjunction with grief, sadness, and guilt following the death of a loved one.

You see that a positive emotion can be used in a negative way even though the emotional intent was positive initially. Through your mental mind, you can turn emotions into the opposite action and resultant behaviour. The opposite to emotional love is hate when you mentally choose to reverse the initial intent. Examples are prejudices, control issues, rage, bullying, persecution, abuse, etc. Many people have these negative aspects of love hidden in their characteristic patterns of behaviour. To this day, I am shocked at people's deep-down prejudices and beliefs. They admit to them, but in the next sentence cannot understand their issues regarding lack of love in their life. With the level of outwardly directed hatred, they need to accept their deep-down issues with worthiness in order to love themselves, to love others, and to be loved by others. A mirror is a very powerful tool for the practitioner to display at this point.

Another common love aspect that holds people back is the story of '**the Shadow of Possibilities**'.

This aspect of love relates to 'the blame game'. The patient holds onto the thought pattern of "my life would have been different were it not for

---

1   *Wherever 'God' is mentioned the idea of a divine being or creator is meant (with respect to all beliefs).*

my parents, my upbringing, my surroundings, etc." They peddle a story that they are burdened with their history and the past. Things like: a rough birth, parents, teachers, upbringing, school or town I experienced, job, etc. They can be heard saying things like "If only my parents had not separated when I was young." They lament, and fail to have direction to move forward because they think that they are unloved (and unlucky).

Emotionally/spiritually, the body disagrees as they chose this life and have directed the journey that they have travelled.

Being 'In Love' (Loving involves a spiritual connection):
To be 'In Love' the body interprets that you first and foremost love yourself: emotionally, mentally, physically, and spiritually. Once this energy is clear you are then available to be 'in love' (PEMS[2]) with another person. You cannot be 'in love' with two different people, other than yourself and one other. To be 'in love' with someone else, the body interprets that you have to love them emotionally, mentally, physically, and spiritually. We appear to have experienced this very strongly in our first true love, often in teenage years, but through experience we mentally work through the break-up and move on, having been touched deeply and having experienced that 'in love' feeling, which affects our total body. Sometimes the 'in love' experience can be an *infatuation* with someone even though you have never met them personally or even had any contact with them! (For example, during our teenage/ adolescent years in particular, when we can be full of idealism, fantasy, romance, and hormones.)

When we attempt to move on, our love energy may still be connected to a previous love or infatuation experience. Having found someone new we no longer love our previous partner mentally, emotionally or physically. However, if the spiritual love is still attached to that previous partner then our spiritual love cannot be claimed back by us to share ... but far more importantly it cannot be claimed for ourselves either. If the energy is not clear, we may not necessarily have problems in our new relationship *but* we may experience health problems and symptoms that affect the new relationship.

---

2   *'PEMS' refers to the Physical, Emotional, Mental, and Spiritual energies.*

The result is that we now start to experience chronic symptoms like back/neck pain, bowel problems, bladder infections, thrush, headache, eye pains, etc. These symptoms remain dormant until we have met someone special, with whom we want to share life in a special way. As most patients exclaim: "I have never felt happier and more contented in my life. Why do I keep getting sick and having health issues that prevent or caution intimacy?" Most often they are stuck in the spiritual (and sometimes emotional) energies of their first 'true love' experience. This is an interesting phenomenon when working with patients and their personal relationships.

When the chemistry is right between two people we have a contract of love, which may be strong enough that we often want others to condone it and share in witnessing and supporting it, maybe through a ceremony to include them as part of the family. However, real stresses and challenges start if you haven't healed another 'in love' experience, i.e. you may have healed it mentally but not emotionally, physically, and spiritually. Previous love experiences can hold you hostage, especially physically. As practitioners, we see this theme in patients presenting with chronic symptoms that have presented on and off for twenty to thirty years after a break-up.

In summary, people often believe they have moved on once a relationship ends. This is true of the mental mind. However, being 'in love' involved emotional, physical, and spiritual components as well. The patient may have released their former partner mentally but unknowingly they may continue to hold onto that person physically, emotionally or spiritually and so the body considers that there is unfinished business around love and forgiveness.

Testing to find the issues and then balancing of energies in the emotional, physical, and spiritual entities allows the patient to heal. Most often this makes a positive difference in their present relationship, their health, and personal life as they have been carrying and transferring negative energy from those three components into their next relationship and compensating in their health energy; they were trying to make up for the missing energy in their next relationship – without realising there was an issue.

Mrs T's Case History

Mrs T, a thirty-six-year-old, attractive and fit woman consulted me for chronic symptoms of: anxiety attacks, headaches, neck pain, abdominal bloating/discomfort, and vaginal thrush. She was married with two children and had an active lifestyle. The thrush started approximately five years beforehand, not long after her last child was born. Her headaches, neck pain, abdominal discomfort, and anxiety had worsened since the thrush problem appeared. Various medications for thrush worked well but the problem returned immediately once she had finished them. Various hormonal treatments and probiotics had also been tried without lasting success.

From testing her body, I identified that she had blocked energy at a spiritual level relating to 'in love' issues. Findings showed that while she loved her husband mentally and emotionally she still loved her first real boyfriend (from when she was seventeen-years-old) physically and spiritually. She didn't want to believe that, but I treated her by correcting and balancing her energies. Before she left the office testing her showed that she now loved her husband in all four categories and so was 'in love' with her husband. I have treated her several times since but the thrush problem disappeared within two days without medication and has not returned twelve years later.

In brief, her parents didn't like her boyfriend and put pressure on her to end the relationship, which she unwillingly did. She met and married her husband when she was twenty-three-years-old and they decided after two children that they didn't want any more. This brought up her 'completion of procreation' instincts that perhaps exposed her issues of love and nurture, thereby compromising intimacy.

Twelve years later her anxiety is thankfully manageable as she still has a husband, two children, a business to run, plus extended family responsibilities. Her other symptoms have not returned as she continues to have six monthly treatments to balance her energies.

Another situation often encountered is that patients often say they are 'in love' with someone and ask if I can test them to see if their body agrees with their statement. Testing shows that we may sometimes think we are 'in love' when in fact many times it is a mental obsession; the other three components don't always agree. This is often very upsetting for the patient but when they own why they want this person to love them and vice versa then the healing can take place. The healing is not only with regards to their present circumstance but also deals with the reason why they attracted or needed that person in the first place. In this instance, I cannot correct the energies to complement their wishes. Knowing and owning their situation for most people is healing.

On average:

- Conditional love is predominantly practised between parents and children and vice versa as there are conditions and expectations on outcome for all parties in the emotional and mental realms.
- We love one another unconditionally at a spiritual level as we are family.
- Physical love is interpreted as intimacy, which you should not have with immediate family members.
- Unconditional love is practised between grandchildren, grandparents, people and their pets as there are no expectations on outcomes – they just agree to love one another for who and what they are. Keep nurturing, profiting, and feeding me, and we have an unconditional contract.
- Unconditional love and some conditional love is practised with friends. Friends turn a blind eye to idiosyncrasies. A true friend is someone you can trust and they can trust you.
- A mixture of conditional and unconditional love is practised between couples who are 'in love'.
- Love differs from Like, Respect, and Trust in that love does not necessarily have to be earned – the other three do. You love your immediate family but because of their behaviour they may not have earned your liking, respect, and trust. If something major happened to them, through love, you would be there to support and help them, but you may choose not to be involved in their immediate or everyday life.
- You care *about* them but from experience, you may choose to not care *for* them.

Anger/Rage

Most people consider Anger to be a negative emotion. Anger gives us survival, drive, passion, competitiveness, pleasure, gratification; when in control, it gives us calmness, approval, acceptance, patience, forgiveness, peace, and liking. We use anger to protect ourselves through our survival instinct.

Anger is often a reactionary emotion. We do not get angry with other people as emotions are self-related so we actually get angry at ourselves because we can't control others who we see as having maybe treated us unfairly or unjustly. All too often we do something for someone else in the expectation that they are going to return the favour. Justice and fairness don't really exist. We can choose to treat others with justice, fairness, and equality; however, that is our choice. It may not be another person's choice to return those principles. (NB. See over-responsibility.)

Rage is 'out of control' anger and therefore has a major mental component attached to it when we can come unstuck, causing harm to others and to ourselves. It is great to get angry, but don't try to get even. Control anger by working out its origins and then making choices to change your behaviour around it. Excuses like, "all my family are angry" are not acceptable but are just that – an excuse. It is one of the most healing things for everyone involved to see a person change from displaying an angry/rageful response to a peaceful or constructive response by becoming communicative. This increases their self-esteem through self-love.

Other forms of anger we treat are fury/a feeling of being wronged or criticised/lawlessness/fretfulness or agitation.

While most people would deny that anger is an issue in their life they are usually willing to admit that they feel frustrated or resentful, etc.

Wronged/Fury

Some people just feel that they have been wronged or ostracised, etc. Mentally they have experienced these situations, however their anger originates from the emotions of grief, lack of self-worth, sadness, subservience, persecution, feeling unloved, etc.

Criticised

These people feel any suggestion, assistance, help or reward is just people getting at them. Their response is one of aggravation and anger; they interpret your attempts to help or give friendly advice as you being critical of them and not appreciating them.

Lawlessness

These people are usually very intelligent and try to help others in an over-responsible way. They can also behave in a very contrary and comical fashion, e.g. they refuse to get a warrant of fitness or register their motor vehicle, but insist that it is insured in case they have an accident!! When you point out to them that the insurance is invalid without registration and warrant they become very angry and animated because "The government and the system is ripping them off!" They may also believe that driving at 105kms per hour is their right in a 100km zone or that the 'One thousand, two thousand' rule regarding space between you and the vehicle you are following doesn't apply to them because they "are *not* going to have an accident!" They can be heard saying that traffic management police would be better placed catching "real criminals". Their anger has gotten in the way of reason and stops them from moving out of victimhood.

Fretfulness/Agitation

These people are very irritable, cross, edgy, touchy, and short-tempered. They interpret any question, attempt at clarification or even an invitation to join in as being an invitation to conflict. They loudly respond to most communications with hostility. Usually when they settle down they are very convivial and pleasant. This trait is often seen in people who engage in road rage.

Jealousy

Jealousy as an emotion is positive in intent. We would not wear nice clothes, live in comfortable surroundings, have a nice car, nice furniture, house, etc. if we didn't practise jealousy. We learn and advance ourselves as humans by observing others, how they live, and what they have that makes life easier, more enjoyable, and fulfilling. It creates motivation, competitiveness, learning, trust, love, indifference, carefreeness, and satisfaction. This emotion, if controlled, can lead to the above situations through choice.

We associate jealousy with the more destructive choices that people make like righteousness, hatred, suspiciousness, guardedness, protectiveness, scepticism, anxiousness, possessiveness, disbelief, distrust, dismissiveness, envy, resentfulness, grudgingness, intolerance, malice, ill will, and persecution. You can choose any of these options to persecute yourself by either behaving this way yourself or by creating the 'non-reality' of believing that others are treating you this way.

Another way you can misuse this emotion is to drag other people down by creating stories and lies about them to persecute them. Righteousness, envy, hatred, and scepticism are not very pretty but are prominent in our society.

Fear

This is the most prominent emotion; we all experience fear temporarily, but some people experience it on a continuous basis (anxiety). It provides us with the will to achieve goals and objectives. It promotes learning, competitiveness, creativity, braveness, confidence, daring, safety, and survival (fight or flight). Fear can be used mentally to create anxiety, worry, stress, panic, terror, apprehensiveness, phobias, agitation, respect, worship, suspicion, regret, nervousness, timidity, neuroses, obsessive compulsive disorders, etc. Most people can identify with fear as an emotion as at some stage in life we have experienced it in the form of 'stress' and therefore know what effects it can have on our bodies.

When testing patients for phobias and fears, the largest proportion of patients fear success; not failure, not rejection, not being loveable, but success. (See 'Fear of Success'.) They fear themselves more than anyone or anything else. In other words, they fear how good, powerful or successful they could be if they let their true selves be known. Therefore, they identify with what they do or represent rather than who they are.

Emotional Foundations

These four emotions appear to be the foundations of our feelings and as you can see, they often overlap with one another. You feel Love, Anger, Jealousy, and Fear, however when you 'mentalise' (think out) emotions they become something else and then give us the choice to change it, slant it or even turn it into the opposite. This all changes our behaviour with regards to how we see others see us, and eventually (if challenged) how we see ourselves.

Emotions originate from three distinct areas:

1. **Spiritual Source**

   In order for our spiritual history and knowledge to be realised, our body uses the emotional mind to express itself, as evidenced in our personality.

   a) Intuitions and knowing

   b) Instincts

   c) Expressiveness relating to Soul Purpose, the blueprint that gives meaning and purpose to our existence and journey.

2. **Familial Source**

   Experiences of our ancestors are passed down through our feelings about living.

   a) Fear Phobias, likes, dislikes, aptitude, and attitudes, e.g. a small child may be frightened or intrigued by a spider or snake having never seen one before.

   b) Beliefs, prejudices, and bias

   Through generations of our forebears of different ethnic and religious backgrounds and experiences, e.g. historical hatreds that override parental teachings.

   c) Family characteristics

   Behavioural characteristics of ancestors are identified early in young children. They can be identified by their predictable way of dealing with certain situations, e.g. being over-responsible, seeking approval, anxious, self-persecuting, addictive, guilt-driven, etc.

   When working with and treating patients, familial emotions are the most powerful contributor to emotional behaviour. In a family of four children who have all experienced similar abuse/betrayal/trauma each child

may react completely differently to their siblings. One or more of the four children may grow up to live full and happy lives as if the negative experience has not scarred them in the same way as the others who may live a life trapped in the pain and memory of it all. It could be argued that mentally they have been able to overcome their experience, however from a treatment perspective they exhibit that they have not inherited the same aspects or depth of familial emotions that have affected the others. This explains their behaviour and their attitude to life from their early childhood years. This has been one of the blueprint challenges they have chosen in this lifetime.

3. **Personal Source**

Our emotional experience of living is influenced greatly by Nos. 1 and 2 (Spiritual and Familial). We are not only destined to act and react according to our Personality traits (Spiritual) but also to our Characteristic traits (Familial). Add to this a good dose of family behaviour due to beliefs, prejudices, biases, fears, phobias, superstitions, instincts, values, principles, ethnic/cultural/religious beliefs, and belonging, and we have a great recipe of ingredients to give feeling and meaning to our emotional being.

Once one enters cognitive and analytical thinking one has some challenging choices to make in one's life, which are exhibited in an open- or closed-form display of behaviour. These factors are what make us uniquely different as everyone in our family does not have the same personality, nor have they taken on similar characteristics, knowing, intuitions or expressiveness of 'Soul Purpose'. Your personal journey and challenges are just that – personal, often taking a lifetime (with the help of others) to own and understand the process.

Experiencing Emotions

We experience and display emotions in various forms and contrasts as although the intent is positive, the influence of the mental (conscious analytical) mind can display our feelings in many contrasting combinations of positivity, negativity or combinations of both.

Our choices are displayed in our behaviour. We can change our behaviour by changing our choices. This comes from ownership, realisation, living in reality, and also healing through accountability, acceptance, and forgiveness, which helps bring about happiness and freedom.

If these emotional combinations stay in place long enough we form behavioural traits. Two of the most common are:

1. Chaos
2. Betrayal.

(See 'Chaos and Betrayal'.)

CHAPTER 14

Key emotions
"I feel"

These are the main triggering emotions that destabilise our energies when we are challenged mentally or physically. They can drag other emotions in with them, but unlike complex emotions they usually relate to specific circumstances or events that are easy to identify for the patient. I find these points by knowing that the emotional system is being compromised. Using magnets, I scan the body and head for energy blockages. Once I find these energy blockages I am able to work out what emotions they relate to.

Generally speaking, emotional points are found on the left side of the body and head. One point for each emotion. Mental points are found all over the body and head. Two and three magnets are needed to harness these energy points. When you look at these emotional and mental definitions you will note organ association, i.e. Fear – Anatomical Association – Kidney. The emotion is fear and the organ where energy is blocked or altered in is the left kidney.

This is often helpful for the practitioner as patients often exhibit pain, discomfort or tingling sensations in or around the area that relates to the emotion. In such a case, the practitioner would rule out any situations that need further investigation/treatment. If the symptoms are long-standing and all investigative tests are normal, then the emotional factor that relates to that area is a possible cause of the said problem. If treated properly and the symptoms disappear then one can assume that the problem was related to an emotional imbalance.

CHAPTER 15

Emotions
(Key, Supportive and Complex)

ABANDONMENT vs Nurture

Anatomical Association – Arm pits (Axillae)

(Complex Emotion)

Positive	Negative
Love	Desertion
Support	Forsaking
Acceptance, Affection	Jilting

Abandonment, Abuse, and Betrayal are often intertwined together. They are all gut-wrenching, often devastating experiences as they reflect off our primal instincts of love/nurture.

Understanding, accepting, and forgiving the Abandoner(s), Abuser(s), Betrayer(s), and yourself is a big step forward. Often some sort of counselling or guidance is necessary to paint the picture, thereby setting the scene to gradually move on to thankfulness for what you have learned and for who you have become because of these experiences.

ABUSE vs Love, Support, Acceptance
Anatomical Association – Mid-Brain (Anterior to Posterior)
(Complex Emotion)

Positive	Negative
Protect	Maltreated
Care for	Wronged, Oppressed
Respect	Damaged, Defamed
Praise	Exploited, Misused
Acclaim	Blamed, Put down
Compliment	Ill-treated
Love	Insults, Rudeness

This is a very complex subject and is not an easy emotion to treat as it depends on what the patient interprets as abuse. There are so many questions; what kind of abuse, when and where it happened, the age of the patient, how long it continued, and how many times did it happen? Was it a family member, a family friend or someone else? What were the circumstances? Etc.

As in abandonment, often some sort of counselling or guidance is necessary for this patient to move on, and own, the issue.

My explanation of abuse is: Someone or a situation crossed your boundaries, values, and/or principles in such a way that made you feel degraded, dirty, embarrassed, compromised (abused) and often that someone or situation was in a position of power where they should have been protecting and caring for you. (See 'Anxiety'.)

ACCOUNTABILITY
Anatomical Association – Area behind the ear (Mastoid area)
(Supportive Emotion)

Positive	Negative
Accountability	Victimhood
Pride	Unreliable
Being present	Unanswerable

Perhaps the most important principle in parenting is making your child accountable.

You can ask your child:

"Have you got homework?" – Honesty

"Are you going to do your homework?" – Responsibility

"When are you going to do your homework?" or "Give me evidence you have done your homework!" – Accountability

Can we count on you? Or can you count on yourself (to be honest, responsible, and deliver according to the principles and values, that we all agreed on regarding what you said you were going to deliver or achieve)?

You can talk the talk but can you walk the walk?

Stand up and be accountable for your existence, your decisions, your choices, your outcomes, and your behaviour. In other words, be real, and live in reality or in 'The Now', not in the past nor in the future.

Negatives are: "It's not my fault; it is how I was brought up; my whole family is this way. I don't know, I don't care, and I can't help it. Nobody values me. No one told me. Everyone is picking on me. I didn't have time. I didn't get the message. The world sucks. I don't know how to do it. I hate you all." – These people eventually become Antagonistic and Disassociated.

Mental Association – These people have an attitude of, "F*** you. I have no value so I don't care." They are antagonistic and disassociated, believing in no one or nothing, having little or no respect for law and order or common decency. Unfortunately, we are seeing more and more young people becoming a burden on society as they have not been taught that their actions and behaviour (because of lack of accountability), have negative consequences for themselves and others.

You can see how this emotion comes through from family emotions and through family behaviour, etc. – self-perpetuated. It relates to **completing tasks, jobs, commitments, and responsibilities**. You can act responsibly but to be accountable for your responsibilities is another level of commitment.

Phrases like, "I could have", "I should have", "I didn't", "If only I had" are all examples of over-accountability leading into over-responsibility, martyrdom, and approval issues.

By being over-accountable for others you end up being unaccountable to and for yourself. Covering up or completing tasks for others does not do them any favours either as you are teaching them to become reliant on you for their self-esteem and self-worth. They never grow up and you as a parent/guardian have done them a disservice. Parents often say, "I didn't have that as a child or adolescent so I don't want them to miss out!!"

Harold's Case History

A fifty-nine-year-old, Harold, agreed to a consultation with me. Actually, he was threatened and coerced by his immediate family.

He presented with problems of breathing, hyperventilation, low energy, mood swings, anxiety, depression, binge drinking, sore mid and lower back, sore knees, uncontrolled anger and aggression towards family (physically and mentally), headaches, and prostate problems.

He would stay up until 2 or 3am playing games on the internet. He had been unemployed for ten years but couldn't be bothered even to mow the lawn. He was totally uncooperative, drove when drunk, and always wanted to be centre of attention at family events. Listening to music was his only joy. He was taking medication for anxiety and depression. Harold was a very big man, muscular and fit, and he looked capable of doing a good day's physical work.

Testing showed dehydration issues, which were helped by getting him to take a magnesium formula along with advising him to increase his water intake. Otherwise he appeared physically and structurally unremarkable.

Emotional and spiritual energy showed as extremely low. Harold agreed that he would cooperate and attend my practice for five treatments. Initially

I had to neutralise his antidepressant medication as it was causing side effects, but I was able to treat and alleviate those effects. We also discussed his alcohol intake and how that would be affecting the absorption of his antidepressant medications. These patient types are always adamant that their doctor told them that drinking alcohol was okay whilst taking their medication!

Emotionally I treated him for abandonment, abuse, betrayal, persecution, over-responsibility, depression, anxiety, subservience, accountability, reality, grief, and guilt.

Harold showed the need to take another medication for his bipolar disorder. His doctor agreed to trial him on this and to this day the patient remains compliant.

He had been the favourite child in his family but his mother died when he was in his twenties. His two sisters and brother died when he was in his forties. He was the favourite son, but could not save his family. This failure led to abandonment, guilt, and reality issues which made him unaccountable; he had feelings of "What's the use? They all died and I didn't save them even though I was the favourite son who could do anything." Eventually, through hereditary factors, and circumstances at certain points of his life that allowed him to get away with bad behaviour, he developed personality traits that have made it difficult for him to behave in a responsible or accountable way.

Over five treatments his family observed big changes in his behaviour, attitude, and willingness to complete chores at home, but the patient did not think there was much change, which is usually the case with patients who suffer varying forms of psychosis.

Eight years later I still see him every four months or else whenever the family requests a treatment because he has reverted to his old ways of behaving badly.

He continues to take medications for anxiety and bipolar tendencies, plus I have added two more nutritional products to help him mentally and emotionally. He still has arthritic knee pain (not bad enough for any surgical intervention), and back pain after physical work (muscular). Occasional tightness in his chest is related to emotional issues – his breathing settles down when he is distracted from those issues.

He now works part-time three days a week, and his moods are steady. He no longer shows aggression and he fits in with family and social occasions a lot better.

Reality and accountability will always be an issue for Harold; this is something he refuses to recognise in his behaviour. His family however knows where to go for help now, when before there was the possibility of him being permanently removed from his home. He doesn't see that his behaviour affects others; in his mind they are the problem, not him.

Two years ago, he lost his driver's licence after being caught drink driving. He was remorseful at the time, but only because it compromised his freedom and independence!

With treatment, we can balance the physical, emotional and mental energies. However, mentally we can only challenge patients on their thoughts and resultant behaviour but we cannot change their thoughts and behaviour for them.

This case demonstrates the effectiveness of treatment – providing the patient agrees to follow through with prescribed treatment. Often, after several years of balancing their energies, the patient eventually 'gets it' and changes for the betterment of all concerned. They usually exclaim "Why didn't you tell me years ago?" In Harold's case, he may never 'get it' but his family are able to relax in his company without fear of violent behavioural outbreaks.

ADDICTION
Anatomical Association – Lateral forehead
(Supportive Emotion)

Positive	**Negative**
Caring	Addiction
Integrity	Selfishness

Addiction comes through as a family emotion. To practise addictive behaviour you have to have given into both the emotional and mental aspects in order to form a belief. Many families have members who have embraced addictive behaviours that lead to the whole family being affected either directly or indirectly. If we look at ourselves we can identify addictive tendencies, but it is another step to give in to these feelings (and eventually thoughts) to form beliefs and behaviour that evidence this condition.

As there is already so much information available on addiction, I will only talk briefly about several aspects of it:

- Love is a major emotion from which addiction originates. "I don't care about you or my family; I have chosen to love my addiction more." "I want what I want and I will do what I need to do to find that love."
- Survival – Addiction is part of survival, but it is the opposite extreme of this instinct, i.e. trying to destroy yourself, which is one of the reasons addiction is so hard to give up as survival is our strongest instinct. From mentalising, the addiction is as strong as survival is.
- Persecution – self-destruction and no one cares.
- Accountability – **Addictive people are usually very intelligent and are always great liars.** They actually play games with their lies by telling one person something and another person something else. This is a trait I often see in children and young adults; observing this gives the practitioner a clue to check for addiction in the emotional and mental areas. (See 'Accountability'.)

"Addicted people don't have friends; they have hostages."
(Unknown)

- Controlling and punishing others (such as family) – they challenge beliefs and standards by choosing an unhealthy lifestyle through substance abuse; porn, sex, cyber and gambling addictions; or cult beliefs. "I will bring you down to size as you think you are better than me."

"Addiction doesn't kill the addict; it kills the family, children,
and people who love them and try to help."
(Unknown)

This is a difficult area once the person has made the choice to give in to their addictive behaviour. If applicable, treatment hopefully prevents the energy shift in that direction in children and young adults. Parents find it helpful to know and watch for symptoms and signs of behaviour that point to this tendency. One of the key behaviours is to 'conquer by dividing', especially the dividing of parents. This is why parents must have an agreement to both follow the same protocol of standards and values, being united in their delivery of rules, regulations, and punishment. United parents are a strong deterrent to addictive children as they cannot get between Mum and Dad nor can they negotiate their behaviour differently with either of them.

ANGER/RAGE
Anatomical Association – Jaw and Tongue Area
(Supportive Emotion)

Positive	Negative
Anger	Temper
Passion	Fury
Survival	Irritability
Pleasure	Outrage
Peace	Antagonistic
Patience	Rage
Calm	Frustration, Agitation

This emotion is actually a great friend and asset, but when mentalised can turn into a great negative. It is good to feel angry, but control it so you don't hurt yourself and/or others. For example, you can say, "I love you, but when you do and say ... you make me feel angry because ..." We use this emotion daily without recognising it, as primarily it provides survival, passion, pleasure, and drive to complete tasks we have planned. In sport, work, and daily life we control anger to achieve and compete in various disciplines. Every activity feeds off this emotion to complete what you have initiated as a challenge or decision.

Rage is 'out of control' anger. We only feel angry with others because we cannot control them or the outcome of their actions. Nocturnal teeth grinding can be a good indication of unresolved anger – own it, feel it, and work out why you are angry with yourself. Alternatively seek help as understanding and forgiveness (usually of yourself) will heal it. Interestingly in contact sport the jaw is probably the most vulnerable area to target via a punch or blow as it usually brings about unconsciousness via knockout, i.e. the anger or drive to survive has been cancelled by a stronger force of energy putting the victim out of contention and out of control.

ANXIETY
Anatomical Association – Anterior forehead
(Supportive Emotion)

Positive	Negative
Calm	Anxiousness, Apprehension
Confident	Worry, Suspicion
Cool	Antsy, Agitated
Collected	Neurotic, Misgiving
Unfrazzled	Frazzled, Distress
Nonchalant	Twitchy, Tension
Unflappable	Doubt, Suspicion
Assured	Hot and bothered
Composed	Overwhelmed, Uncomfortable

Essentially anxiety is a mental form of fear, however it does flow back into emotions through associations with depression and also instincts of survival, love/nurture, and power. In the mental realm, anxiety is the creation of worry and fear about situations that usually never eventuate.

There is a strong hereditary link of anxiety in families that is transferred through the generations. Children are often born anxious into surroundings that perpetuate the feeling further. It then becomes a situation of being anxious about 'other people being anxious about me'.

In the emotional realm, anxiety is about self-worth, safety, and control issues. Questions and feelings like:

- Am I good enough?
- Am I a success or a failure?
- Am I in control?
- Am I safe?
- Can I trust the Universe?
- What is my place in the Universe? (My Purpose)

These people are often frightened (or even terrified) of God[1], the Universe, and themselves, often due to childhood trauma/abuse.

---

1   *Wherever 'God' is mentioned the idea of a divine being or creator is meant (with respect to all beliefs).*

We always see this emotion as a major element in patients with Post Traumatic Stress Disorder. In fact, their anxiety as a child has often lead them to being victimised, bullied, controlled or persecuted, thus creating their traumatic experience. In other words, they now have anxiety about anxiety.

APPROVAL
Anatomical Association – Hip area (Acetabulum)
(Supportive Emotion)

Positive	Negative
Approval	Disapproval/Dislike
Permission	Dissatisfaction
Praise	Rejection
Appreciation	Left out

People who have approval issues are nice, pleasing, and pleasant people. They like to help and go out of their way to make others satisfied, happy, and pleased with them. Their mission is to have others tell them that they are loved and appreciated. Unfortunately, no matter how much and how often you tell them you love them, it is never enough. They have low self-esteem and feel that they are not appreciated for their hard work, dedication, and endeavours.

Approval-driven people frequently display a characteristic behaviour of 'shooting from the hip'. They are often outspoken, intentionally controversial, and they love to shock people. Behaving like this makes it very clear who approves of them and who doesn't. This causes them to then focus all their energies on trying to gain approval from the latter group!

"Be who you are and say what you feel because those who mind don't matter and those who matter don't mind."
(Dr Seuss)

Often, they experience anxiety, worry, anger/rage, persecution, trust, guilt, over-responsibility, martyrdom, etc. This emotion is often transferred, i.e. if you had approval issues with your Mum you may well have approval issues with your wife and it is often very hard to move a patient on with this emotion as it gives meaning to their existence, their relationship, and often wrongly to their purpose. How often do men marry their mothers and women marry their fathers, still looking to change them so they get love and approval?

Approval in a negative way:

- This is a very strong family emotion and is often used to punish, persecute, get even with (or get payback from) parents or children.

Or

- It can be converted into control issues, dismissiveness, aloneness, and even addiction issues.

Directed behaviour achieves goals and solutions, i.e. schooling, education, captain of sports team or leader of group. Good leaders are approval-driven. (NB. An effective parenting tool is to **temporarily** withdraw attention and approval from the child. The emphasis is on only **temporarily** withdrawing attention and approval, relative to their age and stage.)

Holly's Case History

An eleven-year-old girl, Holly, was brought in by her parents on crutches, complaining of acute pain in her left hip. The pain was so bad that it caused her to need crutches all the time; she couldn't put any weight on her leg at all.

Six weeks earlier she had fallen over at hockey and while she was sore immediately after the accident the pain had eased up a little bit. However, a couple of days later the acute pain kicked in and she was living on painkillers and anti-inflammatories.

Holly's doctor had initially ordered an x-ray, and then she had two further scans because the pain was persisting. Her parents were very concerned that there was a fracture that hadn't been picked up. Blood test results were all normal.

Holly was a lovely girl, attractive with great athletic ability and a great personality. The hip area was tender to touch but she demonstrated guarded but full movement of the hip. There was no apparent problem with the mechanics of her hip, leg, and back.

I deduced that there was the possibility of an emotional/mental issue. Her parents said that she was a very sensitive person who cared for everyone and did her best to make everyone happy. This often indicates a person with approval issues.

The emotions that showed up on testing were trust, betrayal, abuse, and subservience.

I treated her and she returned in two days but there was no apparent difference other than needing less medication to sleep at night. This time her spiritual system showed that she had an issue with her mother and an ex-friend, who we were able to identify through her spiritual system. On this visit, I treated her for betrayal, subservience, approval, and respect – with approval being the major issue. Holly maintained that there was no issue and that it was all in the past. She wasn't concerned.

Three days later there was a marked improvement and this time only her former friend came up in the spiritual system. We investigated further and found that this girl had been a very good friend but because Holly was very good looking, popular, and talented she was seen as a threat to other girls and this friend changed allegiance to the girls who were picking on Holly and trying to bully her. Because of this she felt very upset and betrayed.

About three months later the betrayer moved to another city but returned on holiday and wanted to see Holly for a catch up. Holly felt very aggrieved and didn't want to see her. She didn't want to take the risk of being betrayed again. Despite phone calls between the families and her Mum trying to bring the girls back together, she would not see the betrayer again. It was two or three weeks after this when she fell over and hurt her hip. Physical symptoms usually appear after a stress is relieved or the person has made a decision that is self-assuredly final.

I treated her on this third visit for approval, betrayal, and trust.

On the fourth visit, she was no longer using crutches and her thrilled parents showed me a video of her playing tackle with the neighbours' children, running around freely on the back lawn. The hip pain decreased steadily and after several days had disappeared completely. It is now five years later and I see her for a check-up occasionally. The hip pain has never been mentioned again.

This case illustrates how the emotional and mental system can play a part in pain and loss of function. Holly didn't really understand the concept of approval and betrayal but her body still responded. Everyone was happy with the outcome, especially Holly's parents who describe her response and treatment as "magical".

BURDEN
Anatomical Association – Top of shoulders
(Complex Emotion)

Positive	Negative
Freedom	Weighed down
Light-hearted	Troubled, Stressed
Have ownership	Overloaded, Overwhelmed
Have accountability	Baggage, Affliction

This is an emotion that often accompanies feelings of persecution, anxiety, fear, approval, over-responsibility, martyrdom, etc. One feels burdened with the stresses of life. Anatomically it fits: being burdened with a large weight on your shoulders.

CONTROL vs Controlling
Anatomical Association – Lateral sides of neck
(Complex Emotion)

Positive	Negative
Be in control	Controlling, Restrain
Freedom	Discipline, Manipulate
Independence	Rule, Dominate
Empower	Have power over

To be 'in control' is an instinctive part of survival as we are able to deal with and live in the present, forgive the past, and look forward to the future. It is the pathway of everything that is positive and caring. We have to have reality, jealousy, anger, fear, trust, guilt, persecution, depression, and anxiety all in a positive state to achieve being 'in control'.

Controlling can be active or passive. We are all familiar with active controlling, which usually involves someone trying to positively or negatively control others. Passive controlling can be more devastating as they pull back from engaging physically, emotionally, and mentally. This is cruel behaviour, however all controlling issues are never one-sided. Just as an argument needs two consenting parties to prove their opposing viewpoints, we have to have two consenting parties to practise controlling issues! Commonly one side is active and the other side is passive, thus allowing a codependent relationship.

DEPRESSION
Anatomical Association – Heart
(Key Emotion)

Positive	**Negative**
Peacefulness	Depression
Joy	
Fulfilment	
Purpose	

The feeling of depression is an emotion that most human beings experience at some time in their lives. In this capacity of 'feeling depressed', I am discussing **Neuroses** (the patient knows they are not coping, but it is not evident to everyone around them). I am excluding depression due to organic reasons, brain chemistry, nutritional imbalances, and psychosis.

Basically, the negative dimensions of this emotion are denial and underachievement of your purpose in life. We want to feel we are 'of service', 'make a difference' and 'are of purpose'. In another way – Why do you do what you do? Is it for yourself/personal achievement and what you can learn, contribute, and value, or is it for what you get out of it with regards to what you feel and think others will value and praise you for?

"Our achievements in life should be personal not global."
(Unknown)

Depression is a condition that people don't want to acknowledge in themselves or their families. From testing and experience over many years, depression is characteristically your mental mind being overactive, i.e. you think too much, which in turn depresses and knocks down your emotional mind and your physical body. You feel depressed and experience diminished interest in usual activities; you also suffer helplessness, hopelessness, and recurrent negative feelings about yourself. You are tired, listless, have continuing health problems, plus aches and pains. You experience anxiety, and difficulty with getting off to sleep or staying asleep. You also have recurrent thoughts/words/songs that continually run through your head making it difficult to concentrate; your mental mind is overactive.

There is usually a strong hereditary history of this in certain families, often unrecognised, undiagnosed, and untreated.

EMPATHY vs Play down/minimise
Anatomical Association – Back of neck area
(Complex Emotion)

Positive	**Negative**
Understanding	Lack of understanding
Feeling for	Lack of feeling
Appreciation of	Lack of appreciation
Compassion for	Lack of compassion
Rapport with	Lack of rapport
Commiseration for	Lack of commiseration
Warm	Cold

Sympathy is to acknowledge and recognise someone who is suffering from grief, pain, sadness, etc. and to give them comfort. Empathy is a deeper level; it is where we have been through the same or a similar situation and we personally feel their suffering from grief, pain, sadness, etc. There is an emotional point for empathy, but I have been unable to find one for sympathy so far.

A deeper level again of this emotion is compassion, whereby through empathy we actually support and help victims to **heal through teaching and leadership**. With compassion, you give them the opportunity to change their world and circumstances.

FEAR
Anatomical Association – Left kidney
(Key Emotion)

Positive	Negative
Fearless	Fearful, Anxiety
Intrepid	Frightened
Confident	Terrified, Petrified

Fear is probably the most identifiable emotion. We often don't like to admit to fear, but it is a driving force in our lives in order to get the job done, e.g. what would happen if we didn't get out of bed in the morning, didn't go to work, didn't get a project done, didn't do daily exercise, didn't attend meetings, etc.?

We are challenged by fear, which gives us choices to learn from. If it is not fearful it is not a challenge and therefore lacks excitement and purpose.

The problem with fear is that when we over-identify with it, it starts to control our life, becoming a constant issue that leads to fearfulness, worry, anxiety/depression, lack of reality and accountability. **Mentalisation (or thinking out) of fear means that fear has now become a mental thought process rather than an emotion.**

Interestingly a lot of people who are driven by forms of fear are parachutists, pilots of small aircraft, or are employed in risk-taking occupations. The thrill of performing the task safely and competently gives them the endorphin rush that satisfies their emotional predominance.

Fear drives Approval issues in nice, caring people. Severity of fear graduates from Fear > Nervousness > Anxiety > Frightened > Terrified > Petrified.

Frightened – *Wing bones/Shoulder blades (Scapulae)*

Frightened people are great worriers and appear outwardly as nervous individuals. Generally, they live their lives in an orderly/regimented way – to the point of obsessiveness. They have set times, set formats, and set patterns and look out for anyone who disturbs or attempts to change the structure of their routines.

Self-contained, self-reliant, self-disciplined, and self-judgemental, they can't understand why everyone else is not the same way as them (they are intolerant and aloof).

Trust is a major issue; trust in themselves, and/or trust in others. This trust issue or behaviour stems from their fear-formed beliefs. Because of their overriding condition/complex, they disguise their fear by behaving in a righteous manner and if pushed into the limelight they can become confrontational as a way of masking their issue.

The emotional point on the body for frightened people is the scapula area (back of shoulder or wing bone) so over a period of time they appear to be round shouldered and eventually stooped forward in posture. This condition is often seen in older men and women who are busy people, continually cleaning, tidying, scrubbing, in an attempt to make their patch a perfect place for them and others to admire. They relax by reading, playing games to keep their mind active, and continually keep on top of current news/events. Socially they dislike larger gatherings of people but are comfortable with one-to-one situations or very small groups. People generally frighten them so often they would prefer to be left alone, minding their own business. However, it is still important to them that they are admired and respected by the rest of society.

The frightened condition originates from emotional/mental experiences from early childhood and over the years; they have moved past fear and anxiety into a complete lack of trust in their surroundings. Other prominent emotions are: jealousy/righteousness, subservience, anger, shame, sadness, and respect.

Terrified – *Elbows*

Terrified people exhibit uniquely interesting behaviours. Characteristically they are 'dare devils', lack fear and the fear of consequences; they prove hard to control, especially in early childhood. They appear very anxious and unresponsive to instructions. They don't listen but are intelligent and give you back as good as you give them often with the same words, attitudes, and dialogues you used to communicate with them.

Typically, as a child they are anxious about going to bed, staying in bed, and having the light turned out when they are asleep. They show a number of anxieties: separation, environmental (wind, rain, thunder, lightning), social, performance, etc. but are lacking in fears of being hurt or punished (often exhibiting a high pain tolerance to accidents or injury; recovering quickly to fight on). Other symptoms are: unable to get to sleep, constant energy/ activity, fast-talking, over-intelligent, over-enthusiastic/zealous, and most of all over-willing to please.

You cannot treat these people initially for 'Fear'; you have to treat them first for 'Terrified'.

They are often confused by instructions coming from authority, doing completely the opposite to what has been requested. When they are reprimanded, they don't understand; they look at you blankly and in disbelief. Failing to accept or comprehend punishment, they interpret it as 'being picked on' by parents, teachers, and instructors, who all in turn see them as being stubborn, irresponsible, troublemaking, sneaky, difficult, inattentive, etc. This results in behaviour displays of emotions such as victimhood, persecution, reflecting outwardly as outright insolence and anger/rage as they feel misunderstood and unappreciated.

Being terrified is not knowing what to do or say to please yourself or others. Fear has been transformed over previous generations to become actualised into terrifying anxiety in the mind and body.

Eventually communication becomes an issue; these children can end up preferring hardly to talk at all in case they are criticised. Testing shows that this condition originates from a spiritual/emotional fault, inherited from one or both sides of their family.

Adults also display similar behaviours but because of mental/analytical overlays they are subtler, becoming quick-witted, humorous, very busy (mentally and physically). They are attracted to any activity that is seen as fear-provoking like parachuting, bungee jumping, rock climbing, caving, etc. Being forceful with their ideas/opinions, they are fiercely independent, competitive, always wanting the last word on most topics (as a form of control). Usually they are leaders but poor facilitators or supporters as they find it difficult to work in with others' ideas – and because of their lack of fear they think they can do anything without any thought of danger or consequence. Academically they are very bright but only do the minimum to get through unless they are interested in the topic, in which case, they become exceptional and/or obsessed. The best release for them is physical activity and sports, after which they relax and sleep well.

Being close to terrified people is sad for friends and family as having known them for years they understand how they react in non-pressured situations (i.e. off the playing field). Stubbornness and anger get in the way of them being able to compromise and thereby find a way out of their incessantly confrontational way of being. Along with trust, they have also blended anger into their terrified behaviour.

The emotional point on the body for terrified people is the elbow(s). This pain can travel up to the shoulders and/or down to the wrists and thumbs, often waking the patient from their sleep. As children, they often complain of sore tummies, and are prone to constipation, headaches, exhaustion for no reason, irritability, hyperactivity, and also constant inquisitiveness and fiddling – both to the point of being annoying to others in their presence.

Petrified – *Forearms and hands*

Petrified people are often very successful in whatever they do in life – in business, sport, artistry, music, etc. History shows them to be good students and workers but they never acknowledge their success or see themselves as being as successful as others see them.

Motivation is not a problem but direction is, in that they don't know what career path is best. While they are often very successful in whatever they do they often end up in jobs that are way below their ability and talents. This leads to them being dissatisfied with who they are and what they have become as they seem unable to feel passionate and/or excited enough to follow their dreams.

Typically, they do well in studies at school or university during the year but go blank in the exam room even though they know the subject material well. At sport, they show all the skills/ability needed to become a superstar but when challenged and put under pressure they fail to excel, often losing the plot, with disastrous results.

Loved ones back them in their abilities but they can't seem to believe in themselves, which brings about extremely low self-worth.

Because of the level of fear previously experienced in life, their emotions are locked up and suppressed so they can only express fear as mental anxiety. When challenged, they are unable to access their spiritual/emotional side; they cannot feel out the situation as it is blocked. Instead they become petrified, 'cast into stone', and can only express themselves in total panic or anger. An alternative way of behaving is to distract others by becoming an exhibitionist, which later further complicates their feelings of inadequacy.

After the challenge of an exam or game they almost explode with knowledge and skills, often in frustration and/or remorse. If only they had been in control of their emotions at the time when they needed to be. They pass their exams as they are good students but the results are not as good as they are capable of.

They are the protectors of people and society, being great defenders of justice/fairness based on good values and principles. Because of this they are no strangers to confrontation and conflict; swimming against the tide is normal for them. Conspiracists are often born from being this way over time.

Emotional points on the body are the hands, fingers, and thumbs. Symptoms are varied and complex as their energy has been distributed into love/hate, sadness, shame, pride, persecution, etc.

Petrified people are good at contact sports, martial arts, boxing, wrestling, etc. as they don't feel pain like the average person; they are seemingly unaffected by traumatic, painful blows to the body and head. When they are mentally focused, they are real warriors but differ from elite athletes and students who can focus mentally on-the-job and then turn their mental energy into an 'instinctive' level to produce outstanding sporting and academic achievements.

If you ask elite sports persons, musicians or artists how they produced what they did, they don't know – it just comes naturally to them – instinctively. They say they were in a 'zone' at the time and it just happened without planning.

In contrast, a petrified person can tell you all about what they were thinking at the time and all the options they were considering. This leads to their demise. Instead of mentally turning their energy into instincts, they overthink the situation, over-controlling their mind-energy into trust, approval, persecution, anger, self-hatred, and self-pity.

> *"The better the athlete, the more time they appear to have to complete their skills instinctively." (They don't engage the mental mind and analyse their actions; they don't hesitate.)*
> *(Bryan Hale)*

FORGIVENESS vs Blame
Anatomical Association – Top of head
(Complex Emotion)

Positive	Negative
Excuse, Pardon	Long-suffering
Absolve, Acquittal	Grudge-bearing
Mercy	Victimhood
Absolution	Ungrateful
Amnesty	Ungracious
Bury the hatchet	Intolerant
Bear no malice towards	Malice

This emotion comes up in almost every case, but only later on in treatment. To forgive is a very healing experience which makes us feel lighter, brighter, and happier. Leaving the past behind, living in the present, and planning for the future is freedom. This emotion can apply to parents, ex-partners or spouses, God[2], death, and ourselves.

"I destroy my enemies when I make them my friends."
(Abraham Lincoln)

"In order to move on, you must understand why you felt what you did
and why you no longer need to feel it."
(Mitch Alborn)

Forgiveness of ourselves for what we said or did, or for what we thought in the past about people and situations is the key to understanding this emotion. Often when parents come up in this emotion, patients will say, "I don't need to forgive my Mum – we were best friends." I say, "She died, didn't she? And wouldn't it be great if she was still alive to see you/the grandchildren all grown up!?" That usually brings a few tears. To go through life apportioning blame or bearing a grudge towards others only ends in serious disease, lack of quality of life, and also becoming a burden to friends and family.

"The weak can never forgive; forgiveness is
the attitude of the strong."
(Mahatma Gandhi)

People want justice in order to forgive. What is justice and where do you find it? Essentially it doesn't exist other than as a theory. "Stop it!"[3] and get on with it. (See 'Forgiveness'.)

---

2   *Wherever 'God' is mentioned the idea of a divine being or creator is meant (with respect to all beliefs).*
3   *This alludes to Bob Newhart's skit 'Stop it'.*

GRIEF vs Acceptance
Anatomical Association – Eyes
(Complex Emotion)

Positive	Negative
Comfort	Suffering, Sadness
Peace	Pain, Anguish

As with guilt, grief is only an emotion, unlike most of the emotions that have a mental side. We tend to interpret that we are grieving for the person or the loss that we have experienced, but the reality is that we are grieving for ourselves.

We feel sympathy and empathy for family members and affected persons, but grief will often present as other emotions like anger/rage, depression/anxiety, trust, fear, guilt, persecution, approval, control, forgiveness. This explains why people can suddenly experience ailments related to grief from years past, after a trigger such as a funeral recently attended. The patient may experience another grief that surfaces the denied grief reaction of many years previous. Therefore, grief is the catalyst for the body to have a total meltdown as our system was unable to heal and compensate at that time. The baggage has been stored for so long.

(People regularly hold on to grief about their own lives. They feel that they have screwed up, been badly behaved, dishonest, caused others pain, not saved others, etc. The secret to healing is to own your behaviour, apologise to yourself and to others, learn from the experience, and change your behaviour going forward.)

Kevin's Case History

Kevin was a twenty-four-year-old fit young man who complained of acute pain in his left eye. The pain travelled towards the back of the eye and into the left temple area, causing blurry vision, dizziness, dull headaches, and muscle tightness in his neck. The only relief he got was by clicking his neck himself. This relief lasted for about an hour. Because of neck pain and headaches, he was having difficulty concentrating and also getting to sleep.

He had experienced pain for the last six months. Medical tests had included x-rays, two scans, and visits to several specialists – but they had not been able to form a diagnosis. Treatment provided was medication for muscle spasms and pain relief.

I found that there was a lot of muscle tightness in his neck, especially on the left side, but I could not find any mechanical/structural problems that needed my expertise as a chiropractor. He had been treated by another chiropractor and a physiotherapist over a two-month period; these treatments had included various therapies including neck adjustments. No lasting improvement was observed.

His emotional/mental energies were unbalanced showing grief, sadness, fear, and depression. These related to a spiritual relationship with both his mother and an ex-girlfriend.

The girlfriend identified was from when he was eighteen. Initially he didn't think this relationship was relevant. First, I asked if he had a girlfriend presently and he said no. His reasoning was that because of his work and sporting commitments he didn't have time. He agreed to have three treatments.

On the second visit, we talked about the said girlfriend. It had been "full on" and his first true relationship. He had moved on and didn't think it was an issue anymore. Spiritually his Mum was now out of the picture but the ex-girlfriend came up specifically this time. After the second visit, there was a marked improvement of movement in his neck. Testing showed that he was still 'in love' with his ex-girlfriend and therefore he could not be 'in love' with himself or available to love someone else either. Physically and mentally he did not love her, but spiritually and emotionally he did.

On his third visit, he reported that he had not experienced any headaches for the past week and he had completely stopped cracking his neck. He was more positive too. On his fourth visit, he was finally feeling good.

To understand the sequence of events:

Six months earlier (when the symptoms started), he had met a young lady who he liked but he could not commit to a relationship as he feared that as he had been without a girlfriend for over five years there could be something wrong with him. There was self-grief and sadness and no one could count on him to be worthy of a loving relationship.

The area of the eye relates to grief issues.

Without the treatment, he could have missed out on future relationships in his life. He is a very happy and grateful patient and I see him six-monthly for problems he sustains from playing sport.

Three years later he still doesn't understand how his problems were solved with my treatment, however he solicits my opinion for any health problems he or his family and friends experience.

GUILT
Anatomical Association – Lungs
(Key Emotion)

Positive	**Negative**
Truthfulness	Guilty
Proud	Shame
Innocent, Blameless	Regret
Virtuous	Heavy Conscience

The feeling of Guilt is a great burden to carry, usually erroneously. You may feel ashamed, regretful, at fault, or to blame. Do we make mistakes and are the outcomes our fault? This depends on our intent. Was it our intent to hurt, harm or persecute? Or was it intended to help or facilitate?

After someone has died we often feel guilty for not having done or said something like "I love you" or, "Thank you for ..." This is often evidenced in great eulogies. I have often complimented the deliverer on such occasions and asked if they ever told the 'now deceased' how they felt about them when they were alive – the answer is invariably "no". What a difference would that have now made in your life and also in the deceased person's life if they knew how you felt about them!

The opposite to Guilt is Truthfulness, Pride, and Innocence.

To be 'in control' of guilt makes us a nice person and stops us from becoming arrogant, virtuous, righteous, blameless. However, if we continue to be 'controlling' of guilt issues it leads to regret, shame, sadness, and sorrow. "I should have", "I could have", "I would have", "If only I had known, or said, or done something."

NB. Because grief and guilt are so closely linked, something I often suggest to patients suffering in this way is to handwrite what I term a 'completion letter'. Doing so is a good way to help identify guilt and grief.

This letter has to be handwritten and cannot be written in an accusatory way; the format is, "When you said, when you did, when you behaved this way, this is how it made me feel." It will take two to three months to write as you start by looking at photos and making notes. One day you will put your notes together to sit down and write a completion letter, which will involve lots of words and tears. When the patient rereads the letter, unexpected issues will be revealed to them; they will see something new in the words they wrote. The letter is not complete unless it is at least ten to twenty A4 pages long.

Having written it out the patient can move on to accept, understand, and forgive themselves for their experience. They will feel a great sense of achievement and relief. The patient can then move on further by destroying the letter (by burning it, ripping it up, or whatever feels right). Sometimes it's helpful to have family members/friends or the offender read the letter. However, in most cases this is a personal experience and giving it to others to read sometimes leads to further problems.

HATRED vs Love
Anatomical Association – Under the chin (Sub-jaw)
(Complex Emotion)

Positive	Negative
Like	Dislike
Love	Abhor
Treasure	Hostile
Affection	Despise
Goodwill	Detest
Fondness	Antagonism

Anger/rage is an emotion. Hatred is more of a mental thought or decision that flows over into emotional feeling so therefore you can hate yourself, but it is more often projected onto others or onto situations involving others.

Love and hate are often confused as there is a fine line between the two. Hatred is a destructive thought whereby love is an open-ended and constructive emotion.

HOPE vs Hopelessness
Anatomical Association – Diaphragm (which is the largest muscle in body – related to breathing)
(Complex Emotion)

Positive	Negative
Passionate	Disappointed
Grateful	Frustrated
Thankful	Dissatisfied
Believe, Count on	Doubt
Expect	Despair
Trust, Faith	Distrust
Rely, Expectation	Hopelessness

To be hopeful is to be positive, passionate, have dreams, and vision at the same time as being grateful, thankful, and appreciative. This emotion is a flow over from the mental side of hope so therefore can be a negative experience as exhibited in how we sometimes behave. We frequently give so we can receive (over-responsibility). Plus, if we do receive; do we do it gracefully and gratefully or do we expect or want to give back the same amount or value we have been given to make it even, i.e. if I give you a present worth $100, do you have to give back to me the equivalent in favours or presents? Do you feel indebted or obliged to me to return the favour? Similarly, when you give are you often disappointed, dissatisfied, and frustrated as you haven't received the equivalent back of what you have given? Most people deny this as mentally they think this is not true. However, the emotions often present a different picture.

This is a very commonly encountered emotion. To realise this, and then accept it, is often a good breakthrough in the journey to understanding.

This emotion is closely associated with grief, guilt, sadness, and depression.

JEALOUSY
Anatomical Association – Chin area
(Supportive Emotion)

Positive	Negative
Trusting	Suspicious
Indifferent	Envious
Carefree	Sceptical, Dismissiveness
Satisfied	Righteous, Judgemental

Jealousy is usually interpreted as being a negative entity, however in its true form it is a very positive emotion. If we accept that one of our purposes in life is to learn and experience, then jealousy is the key emotion to help us achieve this end.

Mankind would not have advanced to the level of sophistication we have in hygiene, housing, clothing, comforts, transportation, health, communication, quality and quantity of life if we did not possess jealousy. History shows that civilisations before us such as the Egyptians, Incas, and the Romans were advanced and sophisticated in many areas of their lives; however, it could be argued that the emotion that built them later destroyed them!

We can use jealousy to become righteous or to persecute ourselves or others. However, we can also use it to disempower others by trying to appear perfect either personally or with materialistic possessions. As mentioned in Emotions, it is a very positive asset.

Fiona's Case History
Twenty-year-old Fiona consulted me for relief from daily headaches (starting as tightness in her temples then referred around the back of her head and centred into the front of her forehead), sore neck and shoulders, frequent sore throats, pain between shoulder blades, and skin acne around the jaw line and across the shoulders; she also had a lot of premenstrual symptoms.

Her skin and headaches were her main concerns.

She had tried many creams, medications, and dietary changes, but her skin problems only improved 60% at best and the medications caused digestive problems and increased the severity of her headaches. She was a very attractive woman but quite frustrated and angry about her skin breakouts, which made her feel very self-conscious.

Examination was unremarkable. She exhibited some structural-spinal problems but they did not show that physical chiropractic adjustments would help at this time. The main issues were on the emotional, mental, and spiritual side. She was open to her emotional side being a problem as she observed her uncontrollable mood changes but related this to female hormonal issues.

Her emotional/mental energies showed issues with anger, subservience, approval, fear, jealousy, and righteousness. Jealousy and righteousness were the main issues and she showed that this was related only to herself, i.e. no one else was involved. She was not pleased that jealousy showed up, but was willing to try a few treatments.

Over four visits her response to treatment was very favourable with regards to her headaches and other pain. However, her premenstrual symptoms persisted and her acne flared up simultaneously. She was taking a daily contraceptive pill. Testing showed that she was not reacting to it; however, further testing showed that additional nutritional products would support her hormonal system. Because she was a student she decided to leave treatment at that particular time.

Six months later she consulted me again because all her previous symptoms had returned. She still didn't acknowledge her issue with jealousy. I explained it again and she thought that her anger was more of an issue, especially directed at men because when she was out socially, men "hit on her" because of how she looked.

She unwittingly set out to make other people jealous or envious of her. Because of her presentation and appearance, she attracted men who were predatory. She maintained that she presented herself this way because she was proud of looking good and did so for her own satisfaction and pride. I explained that while she was entitled to have pride and to present herself in a way that made her feel good she unfortunately could not control how other people perceived and judged her and so there were (debatably unfair) consequences to her appearance, which meant that it was hard for her to find a real connection with both men and women.

Hard as it was to accept this challenge she agreed to an experiment to prove or disprove my finding of jealousy/righteousness. She agreed to going out clubbing for one night without dressing up, not putting on a lot of makeup, but just going with a casual look. She reported back saying that she had a fantastic night and danced all night "without any guys hitting on her". She was then convinced that she had solved her problem, but still maintained that she was insecure and that men were predators, causing her problems.

As she became aware of her behaviour, her symptoms started to improve. Gradually her issue with jealousy went away, as too did her premenstrual symptoms and related acne skin problems.

Ten years later, I enjoy her six-monthly check-ups to balance energy. Because of her past experience, she was keen to learn more about the mind. She is now a professional psychotherapist and is married with two young children.

Fiona's decision to work on her jealousy issues is not the norm as most patients give up treatment early; they are unwilling to accept or acknowledge their behaviour because it may be a challenge to their righteousness. In most cases of jealousy/righteousness issues, they work synonymously together. Jealousy is an emotion that presents positively but can present negatively, especially when the mental mind gives choices for either. (Animals can present possessiveness and protective behaviour but these relate mainly to aspects of love/subservience or over-responsibility.)

The case shows how important it is to mentally own and be accountable for one's behaviour – before the emotional and spiritual energies can be balanced to facilitate healing in the physical realm. Balancing the PEMS[4] energies will not facilitate healing as the mental is controlling the energies by maintaining a strong mindset and belief. By taking over and controlling that negative mental energy the body is unable to gain balance and be in control.

As I have said before: Treatment can balance and heal emotional/spiritual energies; mental energies can only be challenged with suggestions of more positive behaviours/beliefs leading to improved outcomes and results.

---

4   *'PEMS' refers to the Physical, Emotional, Mental, and Spiritual energies.*

MARTYR vs Someone who stands by their truth
Anatomical Association – The jaw joints (TMJ)
(Complex Emotion)

Martyrs are always 'trying to do something', often relating to 'a cause' – so much so that they are willing to sacrifice their life and existence to prove their point. They lack reality and choose to 'live out of reality'. Their priority system is: the cause, or other people come first; the cause, or other people come second or third, etc., and I come last. "I am the least important person on earth, I am dispensable, I am a piece of dirt." Unfortunately, martyrdom is alive and well in our society – not only with Islamic Fundamentalists, but also within most families, and strong belief-/philosophically oriented organisations/institutions.

> *"All a martyr or a rebel needs is a cause."*
> *(Bryan Hale)*

To martyr yourself for the cause is falsely thought to be honourable. In reality, it is not. These extremists usually take other innocent people with them. The difference these days is that the innocent people are bystanders – as opposed to in the past when they were innocent followers of the martyr (and not necessarily of the cause), i.e. being in the group meant that they had food, shelter, and self-worth. The soldiers killed the followers as well as the Martyr Leader. However, only the Martyr Leader was immortalised.

There are two types of martyr:

1. **The Victim Martyr** is someone who lives their life prioritising so that everyone else must come first and they come last. They are true victims and are difficult to live with and deal with as they are very often sick, unhealthy, and excessively reliant on sympathy even though they do not see that in themselves. They give everything to others, do everything for others, never trust others to help or contribute; they prefer to do it all themselves and often exhaust themselves as a consequence and so become unhealthy and sick. They exclaim that no one else cares or helps. Even if you do manage to help them, they will redo it after you, so that it is done properly and to their controlling standards. These people are very difficult to convince of their

victimhood and when cornered can be very angry, vengeful or dismissive. If they agree to have treatment, they gradually move on/change but can only do so if they admit their behaviour. Most extended families have one or two martyrs.

Martyrdom has a strong family attachment through family emotions plus learned familial behaviour. People outside the family see them as being generous, caring, and saintly people. Immediate family generally don't see them in quite the same way!!

> *"Get off the cross; we need the wood."*
> *(In Maureen's words)*

2. **The Righteous Martyr** is someone who has been a long-suffering martyr but has actually made a career of being hopelessly long-suffering and they are now stuck in a behaviour pattern that no one can help with. They have endless health problems and trouble with family as well as no friends. Everyone is a problem and no one does anything to help. They are always negative and talk about everyone behind their back. They do not seek any medical treatment or any other constructive help but instead sit there like a begrudging gnome. They don't want to talk, go anywhere or do anything because they are too unwell and often are very nasty, angry, awful people to be around. They never change or get better and seem to live to ripe old ages to be a pain to their family, but not to friends as they don't have any! Family members often get very upset and offended by such martyrs and it is difficult to convince them that there is nothing you can do other than to treat them with respect; you can expect very little in return.

This syndrome is seen in both men and women but can be culturally predominant in older women.

OVER-RESPONSIBILITY vs Irresponsibility
Anatomical Association – Both sides of head (temple region)
(Complex Emotion)

Positive	Negative
Answerability, Reliable	Unreliable
Trustworthy, Dependable	Untrustworthy
In control, grounded	Unconscientious
Balanced, Fair	Inconsiderate
Self-loving	Self-serving
Self-respecting, Respectful of others	Bullying
True and fair to themselves	

Over-responsible people are usually very nice, considerate, understanding, and accommodating. They like to please and have everyone contented and happy.

Responsible literally means 'the ability to respond' so this type of person is over-responsible, over-accountable, loves approval, and has issues with gratefulness (feels indebted). In contrast to martyrdom where the martyr comes last, with over-responsibility the person comes second. Martyrs are often vindictive and can be ambivalent to love in favour of giving energy to their cause or philosophy; over-responsible people are forever trying to please others in return for love. You put others first and yourself second in an attempt to buy their love, approval and acceptance. Patients with this problem argue with this every time, but it is true. "I want you to nurture me and see that I am grateful" or "If I look after your emotional needs you in turn will look after and protect me." This is often seeded as a small child when Mum says, "You be a good boy as Mummy has a headache today." (Mummy needs you to be responsible for her by being a good boy.)

There is not a mental side to this emotion, as seen in martyrdom but we can see how it would overflow into the mental. Although they appear nice people they are not nice to themselves and often become victims due to their behaviour, as they get taken for granted or used a lot. This makes them very angry, righteous, non-trusting, fearful, and often controlling to loved ones. "I have done everything for you and this is what you give me in return!"

Bullying originates from over-responsibility in its negative form. "If I bully you into being my victim you will look after me and support me" – even though it is under duress. Bullies are committed to being supported in their insecurity. There are two ways to stop a bully:

1. Isolate them out of their environment because they are insecure when alone and not part of the group (worth issues).
2. Stop the victim from behaving like a victim.

Number two has the best results as there is no bully without a victim. You can have a victim without a bully, but it won't take long for them to find one. Most onlookers can see why someone gets bullied. It's evident in their behaviour. It is not to say that anyone deserves to be bullied, but rather that something in them attracts a bully – because they are over-responsible. (See 'Thomas's Case History'.)

Frequently we are asked to help parent-child relationships in which one child in the family is very disrespectful and persecuting to Mum or Dad as an individual. Questioning and observation of the child shows that they are very attached and reliant on that parent yet display behaviour that is demeaning, critical, and rude towards them.

Testing shows that the said parent and child both have over-responsibility as a major emotional issue. The child has picked up the parent's behaviour both hereditarily and in character. The child is bullying the parent (the victim). The parent reacts as they should be the one in control but because the child senses the over-responsible behaviour, they victimize the parent sometimes to an extreme breaking point. Other members of the family can see the situation but feel helpless to step in or help as both parties react angrily to any help.

Correction of the problem requires (with some difficulty) getting Mum or Dad to stop smothering and over responding to the child. They have to learn and develop a stance of stepping up to be a strong parent and not putting the child and their needs first. Treatment during this time is helpful as we can assist the transition, and balance energies related to such behaviour.

Another mind exercise I present to over-responsible mothers is as follows: "If you were on a sinking ship with your two children and there was only one adult-sized life jacket left on board; what would you do in order to save yourself and the two children?" Two answers are usually put forward:

1. "Put the two children in the life jacket, throw them overboard, then jump in the water after them." Problem! The life jacket is made for an adult and so both children would be thrown out of it upon hitting the water and so would probably drown.

2. "The children and I would go down with the ship together; at least we'd die together." Who says that you as a Mum have the right to make that choice for your children?

If one gets past the emotional trauma of being faced with such a challenge then using one's mental mind instead of over-responsibility as a Mum, the correct scenario is to fit yourself with the last remaining life jacket, jump into the water, either with both children (one under either arm) or have someone on deck throw each child down to you once you are in the water. That way the three of you have a chance to survive together. As they say on the aeroplane, "Should an oxygen mask like this appear in front of you, secure it and allow the flow of oxygen first before attending to children."

George's Case History

George was eight-years-old. He had acute uncontrolled coughing attacks that could activate at any time day and night, lasting up to two hours each time. There was no regular pattern or identifiable triggering factors. The worst attacks occurred when he was trying to get off to sleep at night.

He had not been sleeping well because of the coughing and resultant chest pains. During the night, he experienced hot sweats and during the day he was very lethargic. Any exertion or temperature change aggravated the coughing spells but didn't initiate them. He had been unable to attend school for six weeks but instead lay around home in a lethargic state. (He loved school even though he had experienced bullying there in his early years. Because he attended a small community school this issue was addressed early but he continued to feel over-responsible for his Mum.) His mother who is full-time self-employed had been unable to work while she cared for him.

Mum, Dad, and George had all been diagnosed with Legionnaires' Disease about eight weeks prior to this office visit. Their small rural district had experienced an outbreak of the disease at this time. George was the only one in the district to experience lasting symptoms so his condition had created a lot of stress and worry for his family. Numerous visits to his GP, courses of antibiotics, medications plus tests from a paediatrician had not improved his condition. As he was not responding to conservative treatment, his Mum was giving him several vitamin-mineral-herbal-based tablets to try and boost his immune system.

He appeared happy, robust, physically strong and in good physical condition. He was attentive, polite, motivated to get better but emotionally sensitive. Testing showed his physical and emotional levels were low but his mental levels were high with anxiety.

On the first visit, I treated him for physical infection with three different homeopathic nosodes[5] (one being Legionella), plus I balanced him emotionally, mentally, and spiritually. His spiritual energy showed issues with his Mum and with an older brother. We didn't discuss that but sent him home with a homeopathic remedy to take daily. The nutritional products he was taking did not show up as effective so he was advised not to take them until I directed him to do so.

He had his second visit one week later. He had improved approximately 25-30%, having slept through a couple of nights with decreased coughing. Emotional testing showed over-responsibility, fear, trust, and betrayal. Spiritually the aforementioned brother showed up as being an issue again. Discussion evidenced that his father had two older sons both in their early thirties; one of them was considered trouble. That son had come to the house and threatened George's mother in front of George and was ordered off the property by the father; this was approximately eight to ten weeks ago. George was very upset following this incident. It was approximately ten days later that George started coughing.

His third visit was two weeks later. He was back at school, having regained his strength and confidence. (Mum was also back at work.) This time he was treated for anxiety, subservience, and over-responsibility.

---

5   *Nosodes are homeopathic formulas made up from diseased tissue, fungi, viruses, bacteria, parasites, and chemicals.*

On the fourth visit (six weeks after his initial visit), George had fully recovered and everyone was very happy.

This case is a good example of over-responsibility, guilt, subservience, and betrayal causing PEMS[6] imbalance. The Legionnaires' Disease was the catalyst that surfaced his emotional/mental energy imbalance (over-responsibility for his Mum). The problem or stress existed before he contracted Legionnaires' Disease. The latter surfaced his symptoms but because of the pre-existing problem/unresolved stress through over-responsibility, he was unable to regain full immunity and health constitution. If he had been exposed to any other viral, bacterial, parasite presence around that time, he would probably have exhibited symptoms related to that disease instead of Legionnaires' Disease.

It is a good example of how children can be fearful for their parents. In this case, it had caused some major symptoms for young George. Two years on he is healthy and doing very well. Because of his sensitive, overcaring nature he will need check-ups every six to twelve months to keep him balanced in his energies.

PERSECUTION
Anatomical Association – Aorta (Umbilicus)
(Key Emotion)

Positive	Negative
Supported	Persecution
Comforted	

Persecution is fear-linked: to prove our worth and not be judged by self or others. We see this emotion as a negative one, but choices can result in positive outcomes. You don't have to act or react to persecution, but instead choose your values and standards as to how you behave. Speak your truth without personalising the situation or looking to prove your point, i.e. don't buy into the situation.

---

6   *'PEMS' refers to the Physical, Emotional, Mental, and Spiritual energies.*

The positives of this emotion are that you have the opportunity to be: free-spirited, left alone, backed, supported, comforted, humoured, indulged, consoled, nurtured.

The negatives are the chances of being: victimised, abused, tortured, oppressed, mistreated, discriminated against, harassed, annoyed, teased, hassled.

We see persecution in:
1. **Pack mentality** – gangs, cults, and certain religious groups, i.e. "We all die in the name of our cause."
2. **Self-worth** – fearless acts or doings to get the approval of others as in martyrdom, over-responsibility, over-accountability, subservience.
3. **Demoralising of others** to make you feel better/to have power over them/ to make you feel superior or better about your choices – often experienced in families and the workplace, e.g. bullying, abuse, dismissiveness.

Most forms of persecution are self-inflicted and self-perpetuating as even if you persecute others it is usually because you feel you have been persecuted yourself and therefore it is okay to persecute others. This somehow equates to justice and pride to get even or pay back.

"Self-pity is not honourable."
(In Maureen's words)

POVERTY vs Abundance, Wealth
Anatomical Association – Breast Bone (Sternum)
(Complex Emotion)

This emotion relates to trusting the process of life, that you will be provided for, loved, and cared for. When poverty is mentioned, we immediately think of money, however, this emotion has nothing to do with money as often people have lots of money but can't spend it. Abundance and wealth relate to having a passion about yourself, others, your health, and your life.

PRIDE

Anatomical Association – Lateral flank of body (muscular space between the bottom of the rib cage and the top of the pelvis)

(Complex Emotion)

Positive	Negative
Self-respect	Conceit
Ego, Self-image	Arrogance
Dignity	Vanity
Satisfaction, Delight	Pretention
Achievement, Fulfilment	Materialism
Pleasure, Contentment	Snobbery
Modesty	Immodesty

This emotion relates to old family values and although it is considered one of the 'seven deadly sins', emotionally it relates to being proud, being recognised, being honoured or not. People often lose their pride when they have experienced long-term sickness and stress. A posture of a person standing with hands on both hips can be an indication of someone either lacking pride or demonstrating arrogance and conceit.

REALITY

Anatomical Association – Spleen/Pancreas

(Key Emotion)

Positive	Negative
Reality	Fantasy
Good self-esteem	Low self-esteem

Reality is a forever-changing picture. No matter what you choose or how you behave, the question is whether or not it fits into reality or fantasy. You can think or feel what you want or choose, but do the emotional and mental fit together? My advice is to run any situation by your feelings first and then run it by your analytical mental mind second, e.g. you may 'feel' like running across a busy street, but when you pass it by the mental mind it says, "Look both ways first to see if it is safe". When you look, there is a large bus bearing down on you and if you cross it may be your last crossing. Because of our family's emotional patterns, one's actions can be misguided as beliefs, prejudice, and bias can play a large part in choices. There are four questions to ask here in major decisions or in other instances where you are being challenged:

1. Does it feel right?
2. Do you think it is right?
3. Do you know it is right or real?
4. Ask a good, balanced, and loyal friend if it is right or real.

If all four agree, it is probably real for now, but remember reality is a constantly changing energy.

"No one cares except you."
"Why don't you tell someone who cares?"
(In Maureen's words)

"Sometimes you get the best light from a burning bridge."
(Don Henley)

Reality challenges our beliefs in that it is easier to go along with the pack mentality behaviour. Everyone else says or does that, therefore it must be okay. This part of our emotionality challenges us by asking the questions of, "Do you identify with it?", "How does it affect you and others?", "Does it fit your values and principles?"

RESPECT vs Disrespect
Anatomical Association – Bladder area
(Complex Emotion)

Positive	Negative
Appreciate	Contempt
Admire	Disregard
Value	Scorn
Think highly of	Ignore, Abuse
Show consideration for	Not take any notice of

Respect is not a right – it has to be earned. We all want to be respected for who we are and what we do, however we often let ourselves down behaviourally by losing control, by abusing alcohol, drugs, sex, language, integrity, etc., but if we learn from these actions and choose to gain control and stay in control then we earn not only respect from others, but self-respect too. If we keep behaving the same way that leads to loss of respect from others, then we are making a mistake that will result also in a lack of self-worth. Conversely, if we correct our actions in order to gain more respect from others than we had previously, then we will earn increased self-worth/esteem also.

If we have lost self-respect it reflects in our behaviour towards others, as in:

- "I don't like you so I won't care for you or protect you."
- "I find fault with you so I don't respect you and I won't care for you."
- "We don't have anything in common so I don't respect you."

These are excuses to persecute or judge others. When patients have this pointed out to them they are embarrassed as righteousness, jealousy, subservience, trust, hatred, sadness, shame, fear, guilt, over-responsibility, and martyrdom are often close by. We need to respect and celebrate our differences as we have unique personalities and characters. Values and principles gain respect on both sides.

RIGHTEOUSNESS/Jealousy
Anatomical Association – Tip of chin
(Complex Emotion)

Positive	Negative
Goodness	High-mindedness
Decency	Intolerance, Tolerance
Judging	Piousness
Integrity	Lacking consideration
Considerate	Feel themselves to be innocent
Virtue	Not willing to really listen
Genuinely caring	Taking the moral high ground
Believer in equality	Responsible but not accountable
Accountable	Self-delusional
Willing to listen to others and or be criticised	Blaming
Willing to stand up and be counted,	Persecuting
and accept that there might be a	Superior
different viewpoint or interpretation.	*Passive-aggressive way as they*
	live by rules and regulations.

These two emotions are really one, not in outcome but in energy. Jealousy emotionally is positive vs jealousy when mentalised, which can be negative. Therefore, negative jealousy can be turned back into emotional righteousness.

Righteous people often have no self-worth; they feel unapproved, unconnected, unwanted, and like they don't belong. You can't tell them anything about anything but they go on and on in a victimised way about health or power issues (sex, money, time, control, justice). This behaviour can exhibit in an active or passive aggressive way as they live by their own interpreted rules, regulations, manners, values, and dogma. As they are not gracious about accepting, they feel it is their given right to criticise others on how they live and behave – especially governments, society in general, people or organisations of power, e.g. police, traffic wardens, doctors, etc. They tend to be conspiracists, agnostics, and sceptics.

Therefore, it could be said that righteous people are often jealous and jealous people are often righteous. In both cases, they are attempting to be controlling of others in order to fulfil their levels of inadequacy.

Passive-aggressive, righteous/jealous people display envy, subservience, persecution, abuse, etc., through acting in a way that invites or entices other people to be jealous of them. This is usually achieved by a power game of using money, power, sex, and control, to say, "Look at me and what I have got – aren't you jealous or envious of me?" Generally speaking, men do it by assets and toys, women do it by grooming, clothes, furniture, etc.

This emotion is not a total way of being but most people have a touch of this as jealousy is one of our primary emotions. The worst examples are righteous martyrs.

On a different level, people can be jealous and struggle with self-worth, fear, trust, depression, subservience, approval, anxiety, and sadness.

SADNESS vs Joy – Sadness
Anatomical Association – Front of face (Maxillary Sinuses)
(Very closely related to depression, grief, hopelessness,
trust, fear, anxiety, and persecution.) (Seen very often in
chronic repetitive hay fever and/or sinus cases.)
(Complex Emotions)
Joy Anatomical Association – Lateral sides of rib cage

The two major emotions that drive Anger/Rage are Fear and Sadness. Therefore, we can say that Anger is our way of hiding or expressing our Sadness and/or our Fear. Our primary instincts of survival: Love, Power, Freedom, Fear, and Fun provide a means for us to achieve purpose in our lives through understanding. If we can learn to understand, we can accept and eventually forgive.

"Joy is the simplest form of gratitude."
(Karl Barth)

SELF-PITY
Anatomical Association – Lower back (Lumbosacral area)
(Complex Emotion)

Positive	Negative
Merciful	Selfish
Compassionate	Self-absorbed
Gratefulness	Self-centred
Sympathetic for others	Self-sympathy
Considerate towards others	Self-considerate

We see a lot of patients who present with acute lower back pain on one side. The pain is debilitating, causing the patient to be incapacitated and compromised in any movement of the body or legs. The pain travels into the buttock muscles on the same side, causing the patient to feel that they need to move slowly and in small increments, otherwise they will collapse onto the ground and be incapacitated.

The problem is partially corrected by balancing lower back muscles, but most of the pain is relieved by treating the patient emotionally. Every patient denies that there is an emotional involvement, but that is because they are mentally analysing their condition. Self-pity relates to aspects of love, fear, abandonment, and anger.

A brief case history may be helpful to demonstrate this.

Trevor's Case History

Trevor, a sixty-five-year-old man, presented with acute left-sided lower back pain, plus referred pain in the upper buttock area on the same side. His body movement was guarded in fear that his lower back would go into spasm. Clinical testing (orthopaedic and neurological) was unremarkable and all tests appeared within normal limits. The left lower back area was painful to touch upon examination.

History: The pain had started approximately six weeks previously, after he had a physically active day; he had been gardening for hours and later went out fishing on his boat. He presumed that he'd somehow strained his lower back lifting something.

Many treatments by chiropractors and physiotherapists had helped but he was still in considerable pain, not comfortable or confident, and was feeling frustrated, as he was not capable of playing golf or doing any form of exercise.

I treated the left lumbosacral area musculature and then proceeded to balance the emotional, spiritual, and physical energies.

Self-pity was the major emotion showing; spiritually it related to his female personal assistant who had worked for him for over thirty years. Approximately six to seven weeks ago he had been contacted by his personal assistant's family to say that she had been admitted to hospital for treatment of an acute health condition. There was a possibility that she may not live. Naturally he was very concerned about her, but deep down he was also worried that if she passed away he would lose a lot of intellectual knowledge relating to his business. Of course, he denied this mentally, but his body was indicating that worry and so a deep-level self-pity was the issue.

I told him that the pain should completely fade within two to three days and please could he contact me in four days to let me know how he was. Ten days later I still hadn't heard from him and so I contacted him myself. He was on the golf course and was very pleased that his lower back was completely better; he felt great. I asked why he had not contacted me as arranged and his answer was, "I don't believe that this problem was related to what was going on in my head." We both agreed that he had a lot to learn. We were both happy that he was pain-free and feeling really good again. He then tried to persuade me to see two of his good golfing buddies who had unresolved back issues!!!

SHAME vs Pride

Anatomical Association – End of nose (This emotion links strongly to family hereditary emotions of shame, guilt, sadness, and grief. Skin problems and acne can be signs too.)

Anatomical Association of Pride – Lateral Flank

Positive	Negative
Accountability	Embarrassed, Conceit
Honoured	Conceit, Disgrace
	Inadequacy, Arrogance
	Snobbery, Pretension

It stems from a feeling of not fitting in, not being good enough, not being accepted, and not belonging. These people are embarrassed about money, ethnic/social status, history of family problems (addiction, abuse, etc.) and personal talents/abilities. People strongly affected by this emotion often seem to be fiddling with their nose and mouth in social situations. Watch for it!

The mental mind plays a big part in creating this feeling of shamefulness. We have agreed that we have done wrong and we need to be ashamed of our past and history (the issue has been passed down through family emotions and negative experiences in our personal life that have confirmed these feelings of embarrassment and inadequacy). Addiction is a common place for these people to hide. Interesting that chronic drinkers often develop blue or red noses! Is it just a circulation problem?

SORROW

Anatomical Association – Crown (Posterior Aspect of Head)
(Complex Emotion)

Sorrow is an even deeper level of grief and sadness. These people have lost all hope, all trust, and all belief.

They are true victims, having bought into the situation and now believing that they had something to do with the grief and sadness. In other words, they somehow believe that they caused or influenced the grief and will forever be indebted and will now have to live with the guilt and responsibility of the resulting consequences. Victimhood, martyrdom, over-accountability, and hopelessness are their calling so they live a life of sorrow, poverty, lovelessness, loneliness, and isolation.

This is a strong emotional/mental way of living often seen in countries of strong religious beliefs where the older women dress in black and behave in a mournful, sorrowful way; a display of subservience and withdrawal. Somehow this demonstrates their guilt for all that has happened in their lives and family. There is a famous picture in Catholic churches of the Virgin Mary with tears in her eyes and on her face. The tears are symbolic of humanity's sins and the picture is titled 'Our Lady of Sorrows'.

SUBSERVIENCE
Anatomical Association – Throat area

Positive	Negative
Pleasing	Bossy
Cooperative	Domineering
Get things done	Submission
Responsible	Over-responsible
Caring	Disobedient
Thoughtful	Rebellious
Accountable	Servile

Throat pain is a very common triggering symptom in acute and chronic illness. People with issues around subservience show ongoing recurring issues with sore throats and some thyroid imbalances.

This emotion relates to issues around control. Either we feel we are being controlled by something/someone (we are subservient), or we are trying to control someone or something else (we are domineering, superior, etc.) but it is not working; the result is them being rebellious or disobedient.

Commonly people are subservient so as to become accepted or included, then when they have gained power they want control. The overriding intention and behaviour relates to, **"Be reasonable, do it my way"**.

This emotion and symptom can be a challenge to remove for patients until they can reflect and accept how and why they are behaving in this way. Typically, these patients have a very strong purpose, knowing, and values. They cannot understand why other people cannot see what is to them obvious and so they become controlling (actively or passively) to get others' attention. Then when heard they try to serve the classic pronouncement, "Do it my way as I can help you" or, "This is the best/safest way to approach or handle this situation". These people are difficult to convince that we are not all equal nor do we have the same talents, understanding, knowledge, and especially the same challenges or lessons in life.

Subservient people are often controlling, dismissive, frustrated, angry, non-trusting, anxious, and irritable at times, but they do not see this in themselves. Rather they see their giving side. They see only their positive intent, however their 'subservants' can testify that their behaviour could often be interpreted as being negative when dealing with loved ones. Their ammunitions are the five characteristics of power: sex, money, time, justice, control.

They are great people who are loving and caring, and want to change the world and the people in it for the better. However, their message is often thwarted because of idealistic behavioural traits.

Look around friends and family to see if anyone has a chronic sore throat or repetitive episodes of acute sore throat. You will see aspects of subservience in their behaviour.

Maude's Case History

Sixty-four-year-old Maude had chronic pain in the shoulders and upper arms. She had neck pain from whiplash five years previously, which had aggravated her diagnosed polymyalgia symptoms. She had had a hysterectomy twenty years prior. Presently she was being treated for kidney issues, high blood pressure, and diabetes. She also complained of low energy and was prone to chronic infections of the ear, throat, and lungs. Significant weight gain and sluggish digestion were also issues.

Consultation and examination was long-winded and complex, but she had brought in her medical history file, full of test results, referral letters, and medications that she was presently taking.

On her first visit, she was treated physically for thyroid imbalance, generalised tissue inflammation, plus I balanced her emotional, mental, and spiritual systems for depression, anxiety, and martyrdom, with martyrdom being the main issue. She was also treated for structural-spinal problems (cranial, pelvis, and diaphragm correction).

After three treatments, she felt better physically – with less pain in her neck and back, plus her polymyalgia symptoms had completely dissipated. However, her general health symptoms had not improved because she was refusing to accept her martyr behaviour. I confronted her on her martyrdom, which as usual initiated a major conflict; she did not take kindly to the challenge! To her credit, she eventually listened and started to move forward.

Her thyroid gland was not working well so I referred her to another practitioner in our office who is good at nutritionally balancing thyroid problems. I did not see her again until she was referred back to me three years later. Her thyroid was now balanced as she was taking a different type of thyroid medication along with thyroid nutritional support. The remaining issues were anxiety, trust, fear, sadness, and subservience. Subservience was now the main issue. She spiritually showed relationship problems with her husband and her four children.

Over the past eight years she has moved forward but still reflects on her husband frequently. Most of the symptoms of neck and back muscle tightness have receded apart from when she chooses to behave in a subservient/ righteous way. She then loses energy and her neck and back go into muscular spasm again. Other than this she lives a good life; she is symptom free; always busy with her part-time work, family and friends; involved in everything. There are still problems with her kidneys, heart, thyroid, and diabetes but all are controlled with medication and some nutritional products. Her quality of life is good.

Maude said to me once that I would be proud of her as she thought that she had finally solved her subservience issue. She explained that over the previous week she had only had one argument with her husband instead of the usual seven or eight. She said how she had stopped responding to him in any way until it got too much and then she'd let him have it with all the issues she had stored up over the week. "I am getting better as we only have one argument a week instead of the usual number." Obviously, the issue had not been solved but she is open and aware when she is told what her body is saying on such occasions. A work in progress!

Subservient people are usually lovely, caring people. We see many cases of subservience, and it is very hard to explain the concept to those affected as they don't see that how they behave is in any way confronting to any of their family or friends. They get comments like: "Stop trying to run my life, solve my problems, and telling me what to do and how to do it. You have many problems yourself – when are you going to address your own health and personal issues?"

People who have subservient issues are very often very sensitive to their environment plus they are very knowing. They don't 'get it' that other people are not gifted with these traits, which results in them forever trying to win others over so that they can help them and make everyone's life more fulfilling and productive. Subservient people don't realise that others aren't as knowing as they are and that they often choose not to be as knowing. This leads to frustration and lack of self-worth for the person with such issues.

In life, we all figure we know better than those around us! Reading this book may help our cause.

TROUBLED

Anatomical Associations – Lateral tip of shoulders or Gall Bladder (Complex Emotion)

Positive	Negative
Allowing others to have an opinion	Troubled, Galled
Consideration for others	Vindictive, Agitation
Willing to listen	Bitterness
Graciousness	Ill feeling
Forgiveness	Righteousness
Easy	Grudge
Calming	Resentment
Pleasant	Pay back
Agreeable	Get even
Soothing	Vehement
Peaceful	Retaliation
Understanding	One has a 'chip on one's shoulder'

Often seen in patients with chronic shoulder pain, chronic headaches (especially migraine-type syndromes) and people who have experienced blood vessel diseases like strokes and heart attacks. Naturally they feel anger/resentment after experiencing such an event but the body indicates that the event was caused by stress or crisis from being angry/troubled/resentful at the time. If they choose to have treatment I tend to find that this 'way of being' has been a life-long emotional/mental issue that they have been unaware of; they have assumed that everyone else experienced the same feelings in their lives.

Gall bladder problems appear to have a familial history. Gall bladder removal is one of the most common abdominal surgeries. Most patients deny they are this way; resentful, bitter, etc., but testing shows that it is created mainly from hereditary emotions passed down through generations in the family.

By being informed about the origin of the mindset the patient can begin to accept that they come from a family with such history. This is not an excuse to continue to hold on to this way of being or to keep behaving this way, but acknowledging the origin of the mindset helps acceptance to surface. Understanding its origin helps the patient understand their behaviour as the mental has been given a reason for the event; with treatment, the emotional energies can easily fit in with that mindset. Now they are ready to own their behaviour and also to forgive themselves for their behaviour towards themselves and towards others. From a flow-on effect this can lead to forgiveness of others who have been involved in the scene of events. Once this is achieved, true healing begins.

A point of clarification: anger, hatred, and bitterness/resentment are often thrown together as relating to one emotional/mental mindset. However, anger is a primary emotion and is self-realised and materialised. We become angry at ourselves because we can't control others. Resolution of anger can be gained through **accepting and understanding** ourselves and others.

Emotionally speaking, hatred is supposedly the opposite to love, so it could be said that both emotions have a strong spiritual connection. However, to practise hatred we have to change this emotion into mental energy in order to project it onto ourselves and/or others. Emotional hatred when energised by the mental mind is potentially far more destructive, having far-reaching consequences. Mental thought-processing has given meaning to beliefs, prejudices, and persecution issues. Anger then is an experience of an emotional way of feeling and acting, which can be practised both positively and negatively. Hatred as a mental state can be fuelled by many mind characteristics – one of them being anger, but the nature of hatred is purely negative in intent. The resolution of hatred is achieved by **understanding** ourselves and others.

Troubled, bitterness, and resentment are all negative in intent as they relate to holding a grudge, getting even, paying back, and retaliation for 'perceived' wrongdoings. The resolution of bitterness, resentment, etc. can be achieved through **forgiveness**.

These three mindsets are very different to one another and present as such when examining and treating the body.

Troubled/resentment is by far the most destructive of the three different emotions, as it involves the experience of almost every negatively expressed emotion, e.g. a reason for events, finding justice, getting even, self-pity, self-persecution, anger/rage, hatred, etc.

In general, this familiarly expressed emotion is perhaps one of the strongest driving forces of behaviour in society. People choose to bury it mentally as it doesn't 'look good' in an outward expression, nor does it feel good to experience these feelings when they arise, however they exist through our hereditary family emotions.

If we bury these feelings by mentalising and covering them up (icing over a mud cake to make it look good), we do not recognise, own, and accept the issues being experienced.

As a result, the PEMS[7] energies unbalance, resulting in internal body turmoil. From my observation, this results in loss of function and dis-ease developing in the organs of the associated emotional origin, plus the interrelated organs and structures nearby.

This understanding of body function and integration has for me been my most important learning towards promotion of healing. From my observation and experience medication, nutrition, counselling, physical treatment, and energy treatment may relieve symptoms but this learning has helped me to understand one of the major contributions to healing.

My formula for healing (Acceptance>Understanding>Forgiveness) is demonstrated here as on presentation patients most commonly show anger first; this leads to accepting and understanding, both of which promote healing. Hatred follows, which usually requires the practitioner to challenge the patient mentally to move towards understanding. Once this is achieved, then troubled, bitterness, and resentment are displayed. Forgiveness (which is the most difficult piece to achieve and own) needs to be initiated.

One can say that these three issues are separate entities but they very often fit together as a way of being when observing human behaviour. Dissecting and treating the individual parts as they 'present' promotes healing of the body 'in total'.

---

7   'PEMS' refers to the Physical, Emotional, Mental, and Spiritual energies.

TRUST

Anatomical Association – Large intestine

(Key Emotions)

Positive	Negative
Trusting	Not being heard
Believing in	Betrayed
Counting on	Doubt
Depending on	Sceptical
Knowing	Beware

Trust is an intriguing emotion. You can logically persuade a person to forgive, to be real, to fear or not, to grieve, be persecuted, feel guilty, be depressed, be anxious, but it is very hard to get them to trust as this requires them:

- To trust their *knowing*
- To believe in
- To count on
- Or to depend on something, someone or yourself.

If you are too trusting you can get caught out, which elicits emotions of anger, rage, fear, anxiety, and reality. If you don't trust, you feel doubtful, suspicious, sceptical, righteous, worthless or dismissive.

Trust issues often relate to a history of betrayal or not being heard. These patients are therefore mistrusting, sceptical, and suspicious. The large intestine is the organ associated with trust. As we say, "I don't trust him/her/ myself – it is just a gut feeling." How often are you correct from your intuitions?

The main four emotions of fear, love, anger, and jealousy all relate to forming issues with trust.

NB. As with all emotions we can project our feelings towards others, but the essence of these feelings is that they are self-motivated. Issues around trust originate from the fact that you do not trust yourself.

Thomas's Case History

In 2012, an eight-year-old boy called Thomas was brought in by his Mum for frequent abdominal pains, which had necessitated multiple visits to his GP. Ten weeks earlier he had undergone surgery for a bowel obstruction; he had had a substantial portion of his large intestine removed.

Thomas and his mother explained how he had been having frequent headaches, night sweats, and sore legs, especially at night. There was little or no improvement after the surgery and he now had problems with food absorption too.

Thomas was missing a lot of school and he was really struggling to cope with life. He was physically in poor shape but apart from that he appeared to be a well-developed boy with a good attitude.

At three months of age he had groin surgery and started having bowel problems after that. His parents had tried eliminating various foods such as gluten, dairy, sugar, and eggs, none of which made any difference.

On his first examination, he showed a bowel imbalance and irritation, which I treated with homeopathy. I also gave him some probiotics. When I examined him a week later there was a slight improvement but he was still getting major abdominal pains, not as frequent but still present.

On the following visit, I treated him for emotional, mental, and spiritual issues, which showed up as mainly trust, but also fear and anxiety. A week later there was a major improvement. He had been sleeping through the night, his headaches had all but disappeared, he no longer got sore legs, and his abdominal pain had decreased by 60-80%.

A further two treatments were given over the next month and after three months it was reported that he had only had a few fleeting abdominal pains. He was back at school and things were going well for him.

Following that I continued to treat him on a four- to six-monthly basis and he continued to do very well. However, two years after the initial treatment, he presented with some of his early symptoms such as loose bowel movements, abdominal pain, and headaches. When I treated him this time, I found that he showed trust issues again as well as over-responsibility, approval, and subservience.

Over-responsibility will most often come up with people who are bullying or (as in his case) are being bullied themselves. I treated him on two occasions for that and ever since he has continued to do extremely well.

Before he left primary school, he told me that after my advice about how to treat bullies, the headmaster had approached him and asked him if he would help other children who were being bullied in the school.

He told me that he helped them by advising them to "Ignore the bully and eventually they stop bothering you; they can't pick on you because you won't talk or play with them anymore." Thomas was proud of being able to show others how to solve such big issues. He said that he was now well-respected by others.

Six years later, he is at high school and is thriving. He is well-rounded, with a good physical body and a keen interest in sports, plus showing excellent academic achievement.

Thomas is a sensitive person however and I am sure that he will need to be treated from time to time throughout his life for his issues relating to trust.

WORTH
Anatomical Association – Lateral sides of head and between the eyes
(These two points need to be activated simultaneously.)

Positive	Negative
Value, Goodness	Worthlessness
Importance, Usefulness	Futility
Status, Excellence	Insignificance

Self-worth comes from our Spirituality, through our emotions, and is challenged continually by our mental mind.

Identity is the key to finding self-worth through Purpose – (see 'Purpose') – and then eventually passion in our existence and life. People who don't have an identity through belonging to anything in particular become negative, lonely, sad, and defeated. That is why it is positive to be accepted into a team, a group, an occupation, an organisation, a club, an educational institution, etc. Through education, fitness, grooming, ownership, job, religion, ethnic identification and so on we feel better about our identity. Therefore, sharing a common interest or passion gives us a sense of belonging and a stronger sense of identity. Worthiness is a very complex and wide-reaching emotion as we can experience almost every emotion on our ups and almost every emotion on our downs.

If we share our interest, passion or identity with other people then our passion collectively gives us acceptance for one another; this removes any gender, social, ethnic, race or economic issues and instead becomes a focus of belonging and worthiness.

Our 'survival instinct' links into self-worth as: "You won't kill me if you accept me, as I too belong to this identity." To find self-worth, we have to find and accept what we are good at. This may include the opinion of others, along with an acknowledgement of our principles and values. We find self-worth in:

- Lessons or challenges that we can choose to understand and forgive, e.g. the way our teacher or parents treated us as a child. What was happening for them? And look who we have become and what we now know because of our experience.

- Inadequacies that we may choose to turn into something positive such as choosing to see something as helpful rather than helpless, e.g. Dyslexia may be a handicap in school learning, but is a big advantage after leaving school. People with dyslexia can see and think outside the square, which is a lot larger area than inside the square! Accept the label 'dyslexia', adapt, ask for help by acknowledging the label, and get out and create and invent new dimensions in learning and understanding.

"Not trying feeds worthlessness."
(Unknown)

- In Yourself – Give yourself permission to choose freedom for yourself in life. Don't accept judgement and don't judge others; **we are not equal, but everyone deserves to be treated equally**.

Many people have zero worth or purpose regarding themselves and therefore transfer this energy into persecuting others by seeing a lack of worth in them too. Lack of self-worth is a very common finding in most patients we see. This varies according to what situation or experiences in life they are being challenged by. **"True self-worth comes from acknowledging our values, not from expecting rewards for who we are or what we have done or achieved."** Understanding this leads to new horizons.

Behavioural traits

Chaos

These people create a behavioural trait from fear and trust issues that literally bring about chaos in their lives. Just when their lives, family relationships, interpersonal relationships, and work are all going well to support them, they may create situations by actively looking for problems or by being suspicious that something negative is about to happen.

If they invite or suspect negativity it will always turn up. To put it in a nutshell, "they are at their best fighting their way out of a paper bag". If they are fighting and striving to survive, they feel safe and comfortable as this is how it has always been in their lives; they've always used their survival instincts. In life, they need to learn to thrive rather than to just survive.

If these people haven't got chaos in their life they create it as that's the only way they feel comfortable. When patients are told that they are a 'chaos creature of habit', their answer is always, "BUT my childhood, my marriage, my boss, my work, my family, etc."

This type of response is indicative of behavioural patterns that avoid accountability. Examples such as, "If I am busy I don't have to deal with anything." "I can avoid personal responsibility and reality, thus creating continuing issues in my life and relationships." "That way I don't have to face issues, confrontation, and reality." It is an excuse not to be present, honest, responsible or accountable. In short, if there isn't a crisis they will find or create one to avoid dealing with their own personal issues and/or beliefs.

Betrayal

To be betrayed is probably the most hurtful thing that one human can do to another. There are various forms of betrayal and many different ways that betrayal can be interpreted too. Almost every emotion can be involved in betrayal issues, either as a cause of the emotion – persecution, martyrdom, over-responsibility, abuse, or as a result of betrayal – fear, trust, rage/anger.

When we work with a patient over a period of time who has a history of betrayal, we eventually come to a point where the body says that the said patient "set themselves up to be betrayed" – as in Persecution. It may have initially been that there was not a lot of choice in their early childhood, but choices have led to behaviour that now invites others to persecute and betray them. Realisation and behavioural change lead to a new life of fulfilment, loyalty to oneself, and an aversion towards betrayers and persecutors.

Betrayal most often relates to issues of love or finances.

Internal
Self-betrayal or self-persecution are the most common form as these people betray themselves, or continually please others, which eventually becomes a form of addiction. Givers attract users.

External
External betrayal is created by becoming a victim to another person or to a cause. They set themselves up by attracting bullies, users, addictive people or abusers. They can't help themselves in attracting and having relationships with such people; it is almost as if they have written on their forehead, "Persecute me."

In either internal or external they never see that their involvement had anything to do with the outcome. **If the only common denominator is you – you are the problem!**

Measuring an emotion or thought is not possible scientifically. No two people are the same in their make-up or experiences in life. Therefore, a patient's experiences, choices, and outcomes are different and unique to that person. For me this has been the beauty of muscle testing (Applied Kinesiology) as you are able to ask the body:

1. What and where is the issue?
2. Can we deal with it now or do you need to be referred on to other treatment?
3. How long will it take to heal?
4. Where and what does your body want done? And in what order, i.e. physical, emotional?

"Life experience, your culture, your family, and your spirituality all have an effect on how you learn your emotions."

(Maureen Rose)

CHAPTER 16

Emotional/Mental chart

EMOTIONAL (Unconditional)	MENTAL (Conditional)
Feeling spirited, passionate, adulated	Analytical, rational, logical
Knowledge by Knowing	*Knowledge by* Learning, discovering, studying, schooling, research, philosophy, memorising, creativeness
Beliefs Family – hereditary	*Beliefs* Self-formed by family influence and self-experience/environment
Values Spiritual/Emotional	*Values* Influenced by upbringing and environment
Self-Worth True values (see Purpose), unconditional, non-reward-based	*Self-Worth* Achievements, success (social, academic, materialistic, financial) (see Purpose), reward-based (Conditional)
Intention Positive	*Intention* Positive and negative, depending on the intended outcome
Practical, realistic, factual	Theoretical, abstract, imagination, experimental, suppose, guess

Growth and Advancement By interaction with the mental mind	*Growth and Advancement* By interaction with the emotional mind
Reactionary from blueprint, instincts, values, to being in control	Most controlling, powerful aspect of the body
Personality Expression of our spiritual soul-being.	*Character* Learned through childhood environment. When people can't cope with what has happened to them or what they have done to others, their personality can change. Personality disorders and Psychosis.
Healing Spirit emotion will always heal if given the chance	*Healing* Can only come through making choices to change – affirmatively
History of your life or what you have learned and know towards acceptance, peacefulness, harmony, and happiness	*Story* around your life. Belief, excuses, contracts, negotiations. Outcome related to reward and how you see others see you.
No negative side in Emotions but can be steered in a negative direction through conscious/ mental thought processes and analysis	*Negativity Side* Can bring about depression, anxiety, hatred, controlling behaviour, psychoses, etc.

CHAPTER 17

The mental mind
— "I think"

There are many books, papers, and articles published about 'The Mental Mind' (which is most often identified as 'the mind'). Our Emotional (heartfelt) mind gives us our instinctive beliefs, reactions, and personality. Our Mental (head-felt or analytical/conscious) mind gives us environmental beliefs and thoughts. These beliefs and thoughts are influenced by our life experiences or what we think of as 'our story'.

This conscious part of our mind is the most powerful of the four main energies we have in our human body – as it can overpower and overrule our physical, emotional, and spiritual energies. We have barely tapped into the possibilities of the powers and capabilities of the mental mind as it is raw-powered, uninhibited, and open-ended, which means it can go anywhere and do anything so long as the physical body and emotional mind can adapt, otherwise they are both not going to progress in learning.

Although the mental mind is all-powerful, it can only assume the power when it is being used and/or is 'in control'. It also has the capacity through personal choices to move into the extremes of positivity or negativity.

My perception is that over the last thirty to fifty years there has been a loosening of beliefs, understandings, regulations, and concepts resulting in humans setting greater levels of achievement and learning. The resultant behaviour is that our society generally has a lot more 'freedom of choice', which often leads to extremes in values like respectfulness, forgiveness, gratefulness, loyalty, passion, integrity, etc. Combined with our identity and sense of purpose being so linked to material gains (assets and money), we witness a bipolarization of society in attitude and behaviour of the 'haves' and the 'have-nots'.

Extremes of severity in crime seem to be more prevalent. However, on the other side, there is far more enlightenment and understanding in those who choose to learn and grow. Because of our identification with worth and purpose, authorities like governments, councils, etc. tend to try and fix the negatives by giving money or assets to various causes. Well-meaning, perhaps – but often ill-informed. Unfortunately, due to bad management, lack of quality community engagement, a presumption that 'they' know best what is needed, prejudices, and superiority issues, rarely do we see much positive change. Throwing money at the problem quite simply isn't enough.

Crime and bad behaviour usually have the common denominator of illiteracy (difficulty in reading, writing, maths), which contributes greatly to critically low levels of self-worth, reality, and values of those affected. The 'system' works well for those who identify with it and thereby achieve through acceptance. However, it does leave a large group who do not identify with our education system and are subsequently left to form their own groups, which are often led by educated or partly educated individuals who have poor values but who give their followers what they crave – identification and fulfilment of purpose – by meeting their basic instinctive needs of survival, love, power, freedom, and fun.

I do not have a solution to these problems, however I am attempting to show how society behaves – without values to guide us. Historically religion, ethnic beliefs, and governmental laws kept the standards of society relatively stable. At times, these examples have of course led to deviance in certain areas that can stifle growth and learning. Governments need to realise that media containing extremes in values like violence and pornography, etc. do trigger normalisation, acceptance, and also desensitisation towards deviant behaviour, therefore condoning its reproduction.

Generally speaking, while there are a few bad people I propose that people are for the most part good – they just do bad things and those bad things are triggered by environmental beliefs, unhealthy behaviour and thoughts that justify their choices. This is a mental process that gives us the excuses to react or behave based on notions such as "this is what happened to me so I am going to inflict similarly on others".

For better results when making a decision, my advice is to go to your heart first (emotional) and then run it by your head (mental) and if it fits with your values and makes sense it will be the right decision. Make your decisions based on values (unconditional) rather than reward- or outcome-based values and prejudices (conditional). In other words, give and receive gracefully rather than because you expect a return or you feel you owe.

Qualities of our Mental Mind:
- Memory – involving recall, retention of knowledge, experience, recollection
- Learning – knowledge and enlightenment, education, research, discovery
- Perception – creates awareness, understanding, observation
- Analysis – forming, examination, test, inquiry
- Development and Growth – expansion, improvement, progress, advancement
- Power – control, authority, influence, supremacy, licence, privilege
- Hopes, Dreams, and Goals – creativity, imagination, predictions, expectations, futuristic, compositions, excitement.

Through our mental ability, we create 'Our Story' about ourselves with regards to:
- How we see ourselves
- How we see others
- How we see others see us (most important).

Thus, mirror imaging our experiences, journeys, and findings in life. This results in a display of:
- Beliefs – opinions, faith, trusting in, believing in, or following. However, beliefs can lead to: assuming, speculating, questioning, doubting, martyrdom, and judging.
- Excuses – justifying, reasoning, explaining, defining, apologising, evading, covering up, forgiving, pardoning, tolerating or overlooking. It can also lead to accusing, blaming, criticising or punishing.

- Contracts – agreeing, making a deal, understanding or treating either positively or negatively
- Negotiations – bargaining, debating, discussing, arranging, arbitrating
- Rationalisation – sensible, wise, realistic, logical, cognitive thinking, reasoning
- Cognitive – reasoning, perception, insight, awareness, comprehension, apprehension, intelligence, empirical learning
- Theoretical – pure, original, abstract, ideal, speculative, experimental, hyper-theoretical, unproven, academic, supposing, estimating
- Intellectual – mental, reasoning, understand, learned, intelligence, mastery, rational, expert, genius, scholarly.

The extreme variables of qualities and displays bring about differences in:
- Psychologies – way of thinking, attitudes, behaviour, mentality, abstract thoughts, and mental reasoning
- Personalities – nature, make up, identity, psyche, individuality.

This can change from your original personality at a spiritual level as through experiences you may choose to model yourself on others and change the way you behave. In some cases, we see extremes of personality change that become personality disorders. Although you still retain your original personality traits, you may by choice alter your behaviour as to how you see yourself – and you no longer care how others may see you.

- Character – courage, bravery, determination, resolution, grit, power, fortitude, staying power, goal setting.
  These characteristics originally come from our family's teachings and values, however they may change from experiencing life with our interpretation of success and failure. Our character exhibits our strength of mind.
  The mental mind is 'Analytical/Conditional' (has to be a reason for, or answer to) and 'Rational' (has to make sense and fit into a model of normality). When we combine the mental with our emotional mind and hereditary body characteristics we can get any one (or combinations) of the extremes in our mental psyche either positively or negatively. Unfortunately, the negative side often leads to symptoms of: anxiety, depression, self-pity, self-

doubt, self-persecution, despondency, despair, melancholy, worthlessness, addiction, obsessive/compulsive disorders, and psychoses (bipolar disorders, personality disorders, schizophrenia, etc.).

The stronger the mental energy is allowed to become the more oppressed the emotional and physical energies become, resulting in depression/anxiety syndromes. The further the mental and the emotional minds separate, the greater the stress level. The mental is all-powerful but the emotional is the balancing energy when making decisions as the emotional energy reflects our families' histories and experiences.

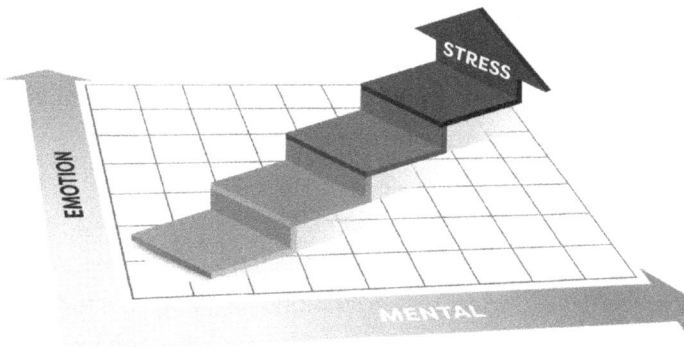

Mental characteristics
Abuse

This has a strong emotional connection but can lead to justification of behaviour and therefore leads to persecution of others. "It happened to me so why can't it happen to you; that way I may be able to understand my pain if I inflict it on someone else." (This is frequently observed when the perpetrator is attempting to understand why someone chose them to abuse.) Weird, I know, but true! Because they are so damaged and have not yet started to heal they say, "I have been abused so therefore I have an excuse to become a victim and elicit money, sympathy, and pity from those willing to offer it to me." In their vulnerability, they give away their power and become a liability to society and family – the 'Poor Me' syndrome.

As difficult as it may seem to anyone who has experienced abuse, when they hold on to wanting an explanation, apology or reason; it never seems to surface. Through personal experience and helping others I have found that the only way to progress when you are continuously walking into brick walls is to reverse the situation and start walking in the other direction. Paralysingly difficult as this approach may seem, I have found it is the only true way to heal this seemingly insurmountable hurdle. If you never try you will never know. You will need support and love but it is worth the pain to get to a place you once thought was impossible.

This approach has to start with an alternative healing way (that involves a lot of very challenging work) of looking at your experience, such as: "How lucky am I? Look who I have become, what I have learned, and having not carried on the behaviour I can now accept and eventually forgive myself for my behaving the way I have since admitting or voicing my experience". Forgive yourself for exposing your abuser and understand that they were mentally sick at the time. Often, they had been abused themselves but unlike you, they chose to try and heal themselves by inflicting the same sick behaviour on someone else (you). Understanding this and forgiving yourself for being the unwilling, victimised person, eventually takes you out of the formula of being the abused. This eventually leads you to come to a place of achieving freedom from the past and your experience of being in a very unhealthy relationship with your abuser. This way you diffuse the relationship connection rather than the experience – as the experience was real. The scars remain but are only painful if you choose to keep giving them some meaning as a way to keep on persecuting yourself. It is hard to imagine that you can forgive your abuser(s) but somehow by following this process of self-forgiveness, it stops controlling your life in a negative way and starts to improve your chosen relationships. The pain remains if you keep on tuning into the relationship connection, as the scars never go away – like tattoos – even though they fade and lose clarity with age!

By following this way of thinking, healing can begin through eventually looking at your abuser(s) as your teacher(s). Your new life can begin. Releasing your pain helps loved ones, the family of the abuser and everyone around you as they have also felt part of your pain along with their sympathy, shame, anxiety, sadness, hopelessness, trust, burden, guilt, etc. Hopefully one day you may be able to help others do the same.

Abuse can be physical, mental or sexual. However, it is the mental that is the key form as the patient wants to know why they were chosen – "Why did this happen to ME?" Of course, there is not an answer to that question but there is a solution –acceptance, understanding, and forgiveness.

Understanding is the breakthrough as if you can get real about the abuser, you will come to realise that they are/were sick and abused by someone themselves. What was happening for them in their lives? Are/were they mentally sane? The abuse happened in the past. Leave it there and move on to 'the now'. Holding on to it and trying to find meaning is a mental decision to become a victim. It happened because you were available and sometimes trying to help or please because maybe you pitied them or somehow sensed their own sadness or anguish. This in no way excuses the abuser. However, acknowledging your place often helps you to forgive yourself by understanding. When you accomplish this, you create freedom for yourself from your past. By being in a position of being able to help free yourself of your pain you can then help others do the same.

Another common contributing scenario I have observed in many cases where patients who are unable to move on from abuse, persecution, abandonment, and betrayal issues is: They mentally hold on to wanting to change their perpetrator, not to gain justice, an apology or get even or even understand – **they want to stop the perpetrator from going on to hurt others in the same way they were hurt**. Often, they have experienced years of counselling and guidance but refuse to give up their quest of being the protector. I usually have to challenge them very directly to "Stop it"[1]. If or when I get them to own their story, they become quite visibly shaken, displaying physical and emotional symptoms of shock. This passes within a few hours, but owning their behaviour is very healing within days as they now know and understand that they were holding on to these old patterns of thinking.

---

1   *This alludes to Bob Newhart's skit 'Stop it'.*

Accountability

Completing and achieving as opposed to making excuses, blaming, evasion, and covering up.

- Mentally this can lead to extremes of behaviour from being: over-accountable for others, e.g. covering up for them by completing their work for them and making it look like the other person has completed the work themselves. This is a disservice to everyone involved. It's all about looking good, e.g. Mum completing her child's homework or assignment or someone covering for others' mistakes or bad behaviour.
- Totally unaccountable to the point of having no respect or responsibility to society, authority, laws, etc. This level often leads to criminal and rebellious behaviour, therefore lacking any values or any decency towards other fellow beings.

People think that if they are accountable for others they will eventually be rewarded; conversely, if they are unaccountable in their actions and behaviour, others will cover up for them. The correct way of thinking is: **I am accountable *for* myself and *to* others. In return, I expect that others are accountable *for* themselves and *to* me.** This mental characteristic could be argued to be the principal lesson that parents have to teach their children, however in my experience it is often the parents who have to live by this code first before they can expect it from their offspring. Institutions, e.g. schools, armed forces, sports clubs, correction centres, etc. promote accountability. Parents are often unaccountable which can lead to their children becoming unaccountable also, which means this trait is passed on through the generations with all parties constantly making excuses for their unaccountable behaviour. When faced with the consequences, i.e. confrontation or conflict they expose their theory of "If I ignore it, it may go away."

We experience environmental lessons from family, schooling, and neighbourhood, which develop into learned behaviour. Through our mental decisions, we reveal ourselves – in the environment we choose to hang out in and by the people we identify with and choose to spend time with. If you are accountable you live by your personal values. However, we see the opposite too where people with contrasting values behave in an unaccountable way.

- If most of the people you hang out with drink alcohol excessively, you won't see that your or their behaviour is unaccountable. To add to this problem, you may be very upset because your children use recreational drugs or binge drink. You cannot preach values if you don't practise them yourself.
- When by yourself you may for example see a gay or transgender person and you are indifferent about it. However, when with all your buddies, you decide to attack this person, possibly causing serious bodily harm/mental trauma.
- You 'drink drive' because you always have and most of your buddies do too.
- "It is all too hard", "When is it going to get any better?", "When will it all end and will I ever be happy?", "It's not fair."

These are just examples of being totally unaccountable and acting or behaving in a pack mentality or in a cop-out mentality.

"You can't change someone who doesn't see an issue with their actions."
(Unknown)

Addiction

This topic has been covered in the emotional realm. In the mental realm addiction is so strong it is often difficult to change even when the patient has supposedly made a decision to change their behaviour. This is because they are prone to relapse and without proper supervision, support, and treatment (medications), they struggle to stay straight/dry/clean.

They have addictive tendencies from hereditary and environmental factors, but it is another major step to mentally make a decision to adopt and live this behaviour. They have decided to love their addiction more than themselves and others and then they transfer that love falsely to their substance or deviance. They have chosen not to stop and therefore their behaviour has become all-consuming – centering around their addiction.

Addictive people use their astute intelligence to 'conquer by dividing'. They constantly lie and even when caught out come up with a countering devious story of blame or negotiation. They excel at separating out, telling each one a different story and as long as they can have one person victimised or supportive of them, their addictive ways can continue as they perceive they still have control over their addiction. However, the reality is that their addiction has control over them, which has a negative spin-off for everyone who loves them. The addict will most often try to cause a divide of values between the *parents*. Sadly, if parents continue to have their values divided, this further feeds the problem and keeps the issues alive. This is often observed in families where children have been able to practise this divisiveness from an early age.

Anxiety

Fear is an emotion. Anxiety is a mental form of fear, however the mental spills back over into the emotion making it a double-edged sword. We feel anxious but our anxiety is driven by the mind being overactive in its search for answers to the unknown. Essentially anxiety is an overactive mind worrying and stressing about every conceivable situation that could happen to us or to our loved ones. The reality is that it rarely does happen but it spills over into every aspect of the body to consume and almost cripple our senses and judgement. It is a great challenge to reality, peacefulness, and harmony in the body as it puts the whole body on edge feeling unsafe, unaccepted, unwanted, and out of control.

Approval

This has a very strong emotional connection and is usually transferred from Mum or Dad issues to wife, husband or partner issues, etc. It becomes a way of eliciting sympathy and attention through being a martyr, self-persecuted or controlling (usually passively).

Approval-driven people are nice people but they have trouble in their personal relationships because they assume a victim role to try and bring about approval. Interestingly, no matter how many times they are told they are loved, approved of or even adored, it is never enough. It appears that they don't hear this praise and choose to carry on being disapproved of, never good enough and not measuring up. They are often very hard patients to move through this stage. If they do hear praise/acceptance they dismiss it by accusing the person praising them of "just saying that to please me".

As they choose to be disapproved of, they feel it is their right to be judgemental and disapproving of others in order to get even in life, therefore bringing up issues around control, subservience, righteousness, etc.

Anthony's Case History

Anthony, a fifteen-year-old school boy was referred to me for symptoms of chronic lower back pain and hamstring tightness. His Mum also explained that he was having problems at home and school with behaviour. He was disobedient at home with both parents and at school with teachers; he was also frequently in physical fights with his peers.

On examination, he did not appear to have a bone, joint or muscle problem, however he displayed issues with trust, fear, anger/resentment, and approval.

Following several treatments, approval issues relating to his Dad appeared to be the main concern. Resulting discussions lead to his Dad coming in while I treated Anthony. Approval was discussed. Anthony confirmed his Dad was the problem. Dad was not surprised as he had heard it all before.

I instructed both men to make eye contact and Dad said to Anthony: "I love you, son, and I am very proud of you for who you are and what you have achieved in life." Anthony turned around and looked at me, saying, "He is only saying that because you are here." His Dad and I both looked at one another in disbelief at what we had just heard!

Interesting result: I asked Dad how it was with his father. Tears came into his eyes as he explained that he had gone out of his way to be a good Dad to Anthony because of his experience as a boy and adolescent. His father used to physically beat him and his Mum regularly, telling him he was a "piece of cr*p". He did not want that for his son, so he had gone overboard to make sure his son never felt the same way he used to feel. However, he was now faced with Anthony's behaviour towards him.

Anthony stood there listening to all this and became very emotional with anger and resentment towards his grandfather. Dad calmed Anthony down and they both cried while they hugged one another. Anthony never knew his Dad's history. Dad agreed to treatment and both parties healed, including the original lower back/hamstring problem. To this day father and son remain great friends.

*My way of explaining this was that Anthony knew Dad was hiding something, which was, as it turned out, approval-based. Through over-responsibility, he intuitively picked up on his Dad's pain and not knowing how to handle it he started bullying and persecuting his father; this was a mental choice as that was the only way, at his challenging age, that he could express himself. **Sometimes the people you love the most are the ones you take it out on or treat badly**.*

Attitude

This is a taught belief relating to how you see yourself, others, and how they see you too. This thought process has strong links to survival instincts.

Depression

From my testing, depression is purely overthinking, i.e. an overactive mental mind. Most people think it is the mental mind that is depressed, but because the mental mind is our strongest attribute when overused, it can go into a 'hyper state', resulting in our bodies balancing energy to send our physical and emotional systems into depression. This results in low energy, poor general health, feelings of being down, depressed, non-passionate, uninterested or disinterested. As the mind is overactive, these patients have difficulty concentrating, remembering, coordinating tasks and thoughts. Sleep problems come from being unable to turn the mental mind (conscious) off in order to relax and sleep. This can present in many ways but chiefly symptoms are that you cannot get off to sleep/are unable to get back to sleep when you wake up frequently. In my opinion, you haven't lived if you haven't experienced some form of depression in some area of your life. It is a challenge and a wake-up call.

Chronic depression is usually a result of multiple characteristics to which you have responded but not dealt with – resulting in major compensations, excuses, etc., to keep functioning and looking good. Eventually your mental, emotional, and physical systems become so overloaded with compensations that your whole system unbalances. In the case of chronic depression, the mental mind (because of the overload situation) starts to internally combust.

The healing of this condition is to have the patient admit and own their way of being. If the practitioner can get them to own the fact that they have depression then the practitioner has a good chance of changing the patient's condition towards becoming peaceful, joyful, and capable of fulfilling their purpose. Once they change their attitude and way of thinking you have a new person who is positive, self-reliant, and confident. What a treat for everyone in their life!

Anxious people can be caught in a circle of debilitating emotional and physical symptoms that make it very difficult for them to change, e.g. inability to get to sleep/stay asleep, can't think or concentrate for more than a few seconds, heart palpitations/digestive upsets, neck and back pain, tension/mood swings, emotional outbursts, and tiredness.

Anxiety, depression, and melancholy are major driving forces that contribute majorly to chronic disease conditions. They have a profound effect on our entire being. (See 'Depression'.)

Martyrdom

Martyrdom and Prostitution, in my opinion, are the two oldest professions known to mankind. One you get paid for, the other you spend all your life waiting to get paid. However, if you don't wake up to it soon enough you will die wondering why you got screwed all your life!

Martyrdom is a way of being; originating from religious beliefs that the more you suffer by giving and serving on earth, the higher the reward and position you will receive in the afterlife, especially if you die for the cause. You may come from a family of martyrs, thereby being exposed to environmental influences in your upbringing; however, it is a personal choice to become a martyr or not. Generally, it shows up in people from lower socio-economic families who have decided to live a life of suffering, not necessarily monetary. They have witnessed the praise, adoration, and control from people outside the family that is often bestowed on those before them who have acted this way.

They put everyone first and themselves last. This brings about character-istics of almost every negative mind condition. While they maintain Victim Martyrdom they cope relatively well with being a burden to their family but once they advance to Righteous Martyrdom they are a pain to everyone and cannot be helped or advised by anyone. (See 'Martyrdom'.)

Persecution

Self-persecution is a decision – where even though you may have experienced this characteristic in your upbringing, it is *ultimately a decision you make* – to live as a persecuted person. This can be either because it gives you rewards, i.e. gaining sympathy and attention – or you chose to be a victim by giving up your power to think and act for yourself. This thought links closely to martyrdom, abuse, righteousness, worth, accountability, and reality, all presenting as a disguised package.

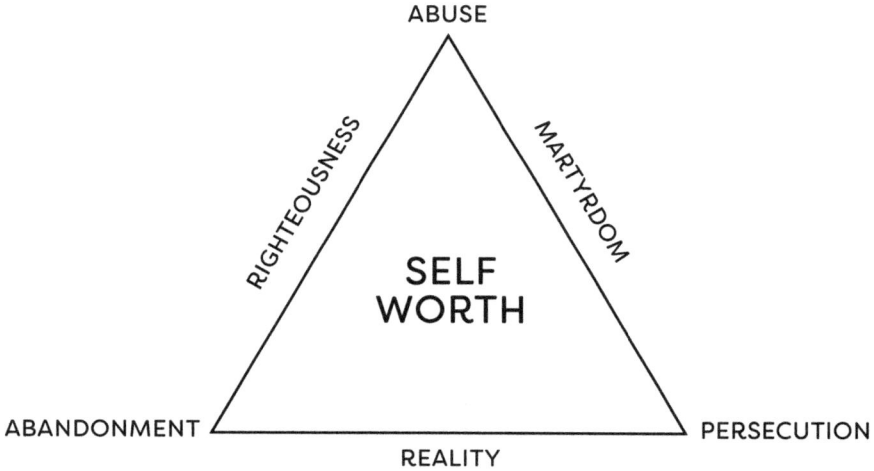

ABUSE

RIGHTEOUSNESS

MARTYRDOM

SELF WORTH

ABANDONMENT

REALITY

PERSECUTION

To summarise, such people think, "No matter what happens I always lose, get left out, punished, woe is me." They feel that they are oppressed, downtrodden, outcast, etc. As you can imagine, this attitude is learned from their background.

Sadly, having made this decision these people often think it is their right to persecute others. They think this way either because they have experienced the pain and therefore it is okay to pass the behaviour on, or else it is a way of getting even with society because that is the way they see the world and everyone in it. They often see themselves as unlucky in life but probably spend more money on addictive habits, proportionately, than those who have purpose and passion in their life.

Reality

Reality is an ever-changing, dynamic way of being and is therefore a very strong mental trait. You may think that you are living and behaving within the bounds of reality but what is reality? What may seem real to you may not appear real to others affected by your behaviour. Excuses like: "I was drunk at the time and …", "She had an affair so it was okay for me to do the same", "Everyone else watches pornography, is dishonest in their dealings, drinks alcohol and drives a motor vehicle, etc." These are non-reality mentally influenced statements. One's values, emotions, and knowing would all disagree.

Accountability, Fairness, Ownership, and 'The Truth' have links to reality. I can tell you the truth now and in two minutes' time (having talked to someone else who has given me different information), I can come back to you and change what I originally told you as being the truth – because the story 'The Truth' has now got a different reality. Often our friends and close family members are best at keeping us in reality and telling the truth.

> *"Level of ownership equates to level of freedom."*
> *"Nothing is absolute or perfect."*
> *"You should only tell the Truth to people who understand*
> *fairness and forgiveness."*
> *(Maureen Rose)*

When it comes to reality, what we *think* or *feel* about something can lead to different outcomes. If our thinking agrees with our feelings about reality, we are probably in a safe zone. However, if your feelings disagree with your thinking you have stress. In other words, your analytical (thinking) mind is usually safer to listen to as it can give you a reason or story as to why you should make that decision. However, your emotional mind (non-analytical/ subconscious), whether right or wrong, can sabotage your decision due to values and/or beliefs formed around that issue.

Righteousness (Jealousy)

There are two types of Mental Righteousness.

1. **Self-Righteousness**

   These people want to make themselves appear perfect in looks and/ or in perceived behaviour. Body image people go to great expense and endeavours with surgery, make-up, gym work, diets, clothing, etc. to appear perfect. They are often unwell as they use diet pills and other therapies and/ or medications, spray tan solutions, make-up products, etc. (which may prove later to be toxic to their body) in order to maintain their presently gained status. They may also behave in an unnatural way to keep up appearances, rarely considering others' opinions or accepting others' choices, preferring to be righteous, perfect, and controlling. Later in life they usually become Righteous Martyrs with no friends, few family members who tolerate them, and worst of all they look old and often quite weathered.

2. **Projecting Righteousness**

   These people thrive on trying to make other people jealous or envious of them. They often look the part in dress and manner as they use materialistic imaging to make them appear rich and famous. They hang out with only the right people, name-drop, go to only the finest restaurants, drive the best motor vehicles, live in the best houses on the best streets in the wealthiest suburbs. Often, they are nice people but think they are a cut above the rest, preferring to judge others by building their own little class system or categories in which to fit people. Essentially, they are snobs and peculiarly enough they are usually people who come from humble backgrounds, have not achieved that well in their personal lives but feel it is their right to be judgemental of others, some of whom are very successful and come from the same background as they did.

   They have often achieved well academically by gaining a degree or tertiary qualification in an attempt to improve their self-worth and status or image, often with no intention of ever using said qualification.

   This thought pattern and behaviour is often driven by family memories of addiction, shame, abuse, sadness, guilt, persecution, and self-worth issues. It is as if they got out of the oppressive poverty trap, having never accepted, forgiven, understood, learned, and grown from their experiences, but instead covered it all up inside themselves.

When you look into these peoples' behaviours, they often have disguised addiction, abuse, and worth issues in their personal life that they are in denial about. This thought pattern is common in varying degrees but often only detected by those who are closely affected by this controlling behaviour.

Subservience

The mental aspect of subservience is that we think we know better than others because we see their situation from our experience and knowledge of life. It is so easy for us to see solutions to other people's problems/challenges, i.e. "they should be reasonable and do it my way". This often leads to controlling behaviour and issues around power. In a different way, some people may act in a subservient way in their family relationships, job, school, etc.

For example:

- You may have to stick with your job and not speak up about certain issues/conditions/colleagues because of the money and position it brings; however, you dislike it intensely. (I call this 'the public service or corporate syndrome' – where you are stuck in a job that you dislike with bosses you don't like or trust as they are incompetent, but because you owe the bank money and you are supporting a family, etc., you are stuck and have to suck it up daily as the alternatives are either not available or are not tenable.

- You are in your final year at school. Everyone has a career mapped out but you don't. Therefore, you think you don't fit or belong unless you come up with a career or tertiary study path that may not even appeal to you. You are under pressure to be subservient in this regard – just to fit in with your peers and the hopes and expectations of your parents and teachers, etc.

Most people would never admit that they are subservient to another as it makes them slaves, however many people behave subserviently to different degrees - depending on what they want to gain from behaving in such a way - whether it be for someone to like them, approve of them, buy or give them something, etc. Situations in life range from 'giving in a little' to outright prostitution 'to get what we want'. The mind will always work a deal to justify it, make sense, make peace, and hopefully remain in control. (See 'Beliefs'.)

Trust

There are very few people on this earth who have not experienced issues with trust in their life. Every quality and characteristic of the mental mind revolves around trust whereby we can be hopeless, doubting, sceptical, wary, etc., according to emotions and environmental, cultural, ethnic, and learned experiences that form our perception of ourselves and the world.

Mental trust issues often result from: betrayal, abuse, abandonment, approval, fear, worthlessness or not being heard. This results in 'our story about our life' – to give it some meaning so we can box it away and use it for any challenge or decision we have to make in the future, therefore forming our beliefs. Sometimes we decide to not trust ourselves and our decisions, thereby complicating our viewpoint by placing trust issues on top of trust issues. If we don't trust ourselves and our analysis, how can we trust anything inside or outside our world. Fear is often the common denominator that forms our way of being, as a person, and therefore leads into any or all the other mind factors.

In order to trust we need to understand, appreciate, own, and forgive how it was for those who were challenging us at the time we made our analysis, decisions, etc. Non-trusting is quite a self-centred way of being as we do not trust others trying to help us, nor do we trust ourselves to change and find a different way of behaving. This often leads to dismissiveness and non-accountability. Trust and Fear are great allies and work together to create 'Chaos'. (See 'Chaos'.)

Worth (Materialistic)

This worth relates to materialistic purpose as discussed in 'Purpose'. You are able to judge yourself and judge others according to the car you/they drive, the street and house you/they live in, your/their job, you/their family, etc. Therefore, there is a close relationship to Righteousness (Jealousy).

Worth (Self)

- Relates to personal matters and standards that you think matter to yourself and others.
- We go on a diet to look good; this increases our self-esteem and self-worth. You may achieve success in relationships, jobs, and life generally but once achieved you go back to your old ways of overeating, under-exercising, eventually gaining weight, becoming depressed with the whole cycle repeating itself.
- Your car and your house always look their very best when you sell them – even better perhaps than when you bought them!
- You may think you need a facelift, Botox injections, liposuction, breast implants, etc. to make you feel better. However, it is about 'how it looks' and is not about feeling – you just think you feel.

A lot of people become addicted to adrenaline and want excitement constantly, therefore looking outwardly rather than inwardly at times of crisis. This is often seen in men and women between the ages of forty-five to fifty-five years when they may experience a midlife crisis and go out looking for more meaning in their lives, ending up in separation/divorce as they are looking for someone or something to give them self-worth, happiness, passion, and meaning. They *think* they are 'in love' with this new person but in fact do not *feel* 'in love' and spiritually are not 'in love'; after a few years, they realise that running off with their colleague or gym buddy has not turned out as they thought it would. This syndrome is reaching epidemic levels in our society as people are looking for a quick fix mentally but are not living or acting by their feelings or values.

Worth relates strongly to belonging and being part of a group, organisation or club with similar minded people. Unless you behave and act on your values, plus find your true purpose in self-fulfilment, then low self-esteem and low self-worth result.

Often patients explain that they ran off from their long-standing relationship or started telling lies to support their deceitful decisions because they were driven by hormones and the rush of adrenaline, resulting in them making unrealistic decisions and claims. In other words, their mind decisions were taken over by the excessive hormonal activity in their body.

Even though this syndrome is well documented in literature and is measurable by blood tests and clinical testing results, from my testing I have never found evidence of this 'syndrome' (of the hormonal system being the initiator of the issue); rather, the mental mind has driven the idea or decision resulting in the hormonal system trying to compensate or balance energy in response. The person has become overwhelmed and feels out of control but I argue that this situation is initiated and driven from the *mind decisions affecting hormonal imbalance* rather than the other way around.

CHAPTER 18

Depression/anxiety/ melancholy

I have talked about depression a lot because with almost every chronic disease we see at our practice there is a pattern of an overactive mental mind – with resulting low energy in the physical, emotional, and spiritual systems. Anxiety presents with different symptoms to depression; however, anxiety is included under the depression umbrella.

In our office, we see a predominance of functional depression – as opposed to pathological depression where there is nervous system or brain pathology (tissue damage), psychosis, bipolar conditions, personality disorders, etc. The latter group are usually on medication for life but find our treatment valuable for balancing their body, which keeps them healthy and able to function in life. We are also able to reinforce the fact that they must keep taking their medication to maintain mental stability and continue to live in reality. In some cases, the body builds resistance to the medications and over a period of time they start developing side-effects. Fortunately, I have been able to develop techniques using homeopathy that neutralise these side effects.

Depression and all its forms is one of society's leading public health issues. According to reports from the World Health Organization fact sheet on Depression (World Health Organization [WHO], 2017),

- Depression is the leading cause of disability worldwide, and is a major contributor to the overall global burden of disease.
- At its worst, depression can lead to suicide. (Suicide is the second leading cause of death in fifteen to twenty-nine year olds.)

- Depression is different from usual mood fluctuations when we observe short-lived emotional responses to challenges in everyday life.

There has been significant research and progress in neuroscience over the past two decades. However, depression is still often difficult to treat, as there is a stigma involved in being diagnosed with the condition and some people experience side-effects from taking medication. The condition involves both the emotional and the mental mind equally, plus it flows on into the physical body too.

In reality, you are not mentally depressed but actually you are mentally over-energised and emotionally/physically under-energised or depressed. The mental mind, being overruling and powerful, has taken energy from the physical and emotional systems. The spiritual system is the white flag waver (surrender) so therefore opts out for preservation, saving itself for another day.

From my experience, there are several categories of depression that we encounter.

1. **Functional depression** – a temporary imbalance state that can be helped, with or without medication and/or nutrition, with treatment of the Hale Technique, to reach a healthy state. If medication is needed initially the patient can later come off medication after anywhere between a six-to twelve-month period. With three-to four-monthly maintenance-treatments they remain in a stable condition.

2. **Pathological depression** – a permanent imbalance, lesion or pathology of tissue that needs permanent medication and/or care for the rest of their life. These patients usually show neurotransmitter imbalances in the brain and/or the body. Usually, we are able to further assist them with treatment and if applicable, nutritional supplements. As they say, "The medication stops me from having acute episodes whereas you keep me stable and healthy." Over the years, with having regular treatment, the number of medications can be decreased (from the four or five initially needed to keep them stable) to one or two. Another comment is, "Now I have a life; thank you."

3. **Post traumatic depression** – this condition comes about by the patient shutting down/starving the emotional system, resulting in them becoming

disassociated, disinterested, disempowered, and unaccountable. They don't care anymore as they have lost their love, purpose, and passion in life. The origin, as noted in the title, is caused by singular or multiple emotional/ mental or physical traumas (injuries or accidents).

If these people, firstly (and most importantly) **want to get better, and secondly are willing to get better (by following treatment protocol)**, they fit into the functional depression category above. Disappointingly, through stubbornness and attention-seeking behaviour, some hold out for a lifetime of suffering and misery, not only for themselves, but also for family and the few friends they still have left.

Most depression cases show familial traits in the three categories listed above. For our techniques to work, temporary medication is often needed to balance the brain/body chemistry. In my experience, treatment is totally ineffective unless the patient has firstly accepted that there is a problem, and secondly has agreed to take the medication and/or receive treatment. A lot of patients and natural health practitioners are anti these medications as they think there must be a more natural or holistic way to treat depression, plus they believe these medications to be overprescribed. I too used to belong to that belief set; however, from experience over the last twenty years (in cases where neurotransmitters and brain chemistry are out of balance), I don't know a better way to stabilise patients afflicted with an 'out-of-control', overactive mind. I am always on the lookout for nutritional products that may have the same or a similar effect but in all these years I have found nothing that comes even close. Nutrition helps to stabilise the condition but does not change the chemistry.

If the right medication is prescribed and the patient is supervised, the effects are extremely positive and the patient becomes a new person. The patient also needs to address and own the factors that caused the problem initially, but without balancing brain chemistry at a chemical level, treatment does not work, as the mind is literally 'on fire'.

A simple analogy is: if you have a fire in your house then you call the fire brigade, not the builder, plumber or electrician. You may well need them later but let's put out the fire first, then analyse and rebuild.

Many people take life-sustaining medication daily to support various body organs. **Why is there such an issue with taking medication to sustain and balance arguably the most important organ in the body – the brain?**

Anxiety/depression

This is the most common form of depression that we see in our practice. The patients are chronic creators of worry, stress, panic, and anxiety situations. This way of being is created by a combination of brain/body chemistry problems, inherited family/ancestral emotions, and learned family behaviour – the combinations are numerous and variable. These patients might have difficulty coping with life, they feel down, have trouble sleeping and/or getting off to sleep, low libido (sex drive), are frequently anxious (about anything), experience repetitive music and words or sayings in their head, experience heart flutters, endure gut upsets, have stress headaches, and are chronically tired or exhausted. They are often too tired to think about most things, including exercise.

Anxiety/depression is seen in people who tend to 'over-please' by nature, so often they need some sort of medication or nutritional support to artificially simmer them down, in order for the treatment to have a chance to work effectively.

Physically induced depression

- **Chemical** – hormonal imbalances occur in both men and women. We hear about postnatal depression and menopausal depression in women, but men also experience depression anywhere from age thirty-five years onwards. If this goes undiagnosed and untreated, we end up with grumpy, frustrated, ill-tempered men, who we assume are just ageing quickly. Often, they are testosterone-deficient, something which can be effectively treated without medication. Men are also prone to family creation/fatherhood depression. ("What the hell is all this about? I thought we were a good couple together. Now we have all these parasites!!") This can be functional or hormonal in origin.
NB. Testosterone: It is not an anger-producing hormone. It promotes drive and action and competitiveness in life. Old men become more placid through lack of drive, not lack of anger.

- **Toxicity** – many insecticides, agricultural chemicals, adhesives, and industrial chemicals, along with toxic metals like lead, mercury, cadmium, copper, silver, nickel, and aluminium can have a negative influence on the immune and hormonal systems. The patient may suffer long-term physical depression, which eventually can flow over to affect the mind as well.

    Observation shows that these people are very sensitive in all aspects of their life, and typically they show up reactions to foods, chemicals, antigens/pollens, metals, vaccinations, etc., as well as being emotionally/mentally that way too.

    NB. Gold and titanium don't appear to be metals that cause sensitive reactions in the body. On occasions when patients experience a reaction to an implant or prosthesis (hip, knee, shoulder replacement) they don't appear to have reacted to the metal; rather, their body has overreacted and is 'in shock' from the procedure or surgery performed.

    Some medications and also nutritional supplements can cause reactions that can lead to physical symptoms and/or depression.

- **Stress and exhaustion** – family, home life, work, and personal relationships are the most common causes of anxiety/depression. However poor nutrition, poor hygiene, smoking, excessive alcohol intake, recreational drugs, etc., are all major contributing factors, by way of the fact that they cause a major body exhaustion, to which the mental mind responds, by taking over the energies required to live one's life to the expectations of the owner. If and when they break down, they exhibit anxiety/depression or post-traumatic depression symptoms.

Chronic depression

Chronic depression is usually a result of multiple mental challenges to which the patient has responded by making unhealthy choices. This has resulted in the patient creating and believing their own narrative as a way of continuing to function and to keep up appearances. Eventually the mental, emotional, and physical systems become overloaded and all systems crash and expose the typical symptoms listed above.

Many people have functioned for years, all the while thinking that how they feel is normal, when in fact they have brain/body neurotransmitter and chemical imbalances; they are suffering from depression. If the problem presents, and the patient agrees to have treatment, they cannot believe the difference in themselves after just a few treatments. Their outlook improves; feelings of self-worth, well-being, and happiness surface for the first time in a long time.

I always suggest that patients have their children checked so we can, if applicable, address it before they reach puberty, adolescence, and adulthood – when behaviour and beliefs become well established. Potentially there can be far-reaching consequences for them, personally, and also for their families and loved ones.

Parents can often spot early signs of imbalance but because they are aware of family history they may be reluctant to seek help as they perceive antidepressants as being the only treatment option. The child's behaviour can lead to the whole family being affected. However, often the child's reluctance to have any counselling or therapy is supported by parents who may be fearful of what their child could say.

Hormonal milestones such as puberty, pregnancy, childbirth, menopause, and relationship break-ups can be major triggers for women. Puberty, accidents and injuries, job losses, stress at work, and relationship break-ups are triggers for men.

Depression is not a condition most people want to be associated or diagnosed with as it suggests weakness, however as I have stated earlier, this condition comes from an overactive mind. It is not your thinking, mental, analytical mind that is depressed; it is your body and your emotional mind that are compromised and depressed, as evidenced in the symptoms.

To me, depression suggests high intelligence rather than mental weakness.

We can experience physical depression from stress and/or illness. Often the body tries to balance itself by compensating; it alters the function and energy in:

- The nervous system (brain, spinal cord, and nerves)
- The mental system (overthinking and storytelling)
- The immune system (inflammatory response).

Therefore, it can be said that depression is not just a mind problem, but a total body problem, and in an attempt to balance energy the nervous system and the immune system eventually break down, sometimes resulting in the body internally attacking itself, as seen in autoimmune (immune system breakdown) and neurological conditions (nervous breakdown). As a result, the mental system stays intact as it is the ultimate system; it takes energy from wherever it can in order to continue the facade of coping. It is not until the mental system reaches a stage where *it too* can no longer cope that we get the symptoms of a 'fallout', indicating that we are in crisis or victim mode (mental breakdown).

Of the many mentally over-energised patients we see, approximately only 10% will need medication to balance them before we can treat them effectively. Through muscle testing, we can suggest the type of medication, the dosage, and when to take it; we cannot prescribe medication. Sometimes GPs question our testing methods and complain that they are not scientific. My answer is, "I test the medication on my patients to see if it suits them, and I will stand by that." It is difficult to diagnose exactly from just a symptom picture, plus the prescribing doctor has to prioritise the options, according to what the various health funders will provide.

In my opinion, as long as the patient wants to co-operate and follow treatment protocol, working with depression/anxiety is pleasing and rewarding. Working with these patients gives them the opportunity to accept their condition, understand themselves and their family's behaviours, as well as giving them the opportunity to grow as a person and teach/help others.

A diagnosis of anxiety/depression does not have to be a burden that categorises one into a state-of-being; it does not mean that you have been cast with a condition that is not able to be overcome or stabilised. As shown here, medication is often just one option.

In my observation, human beings are great adapters to the environment and to the stress of living our lives; however, as new technology emerges to challenge us at a mental level – as seen in our vehicles, houses, workplaces, and personal lives – it is no wonder the mind is showing signs of overload as evidenced in the increasing incidence of depression/anxiety symptoms seen in our society today.

Melancholy *'The Blues'*

Melancholy is distinctively different to, but often plays its role in conjunction with, depression/anxiety. People who suffer with melancholy usually appear to be very happy and joyful, but underneath they periodically suffer feelings of unhappiness, dispiritedness (lose their spiritual identity), discouragement, dejection, and disappointment about everything but especially themselves. They experience mood swings (often extreme) and are therefore very unpredictable to read for family, friends, etc. Often, they are attracted to chemical substances like alcohol and recreational drugs. These chemicals change their personalities dramatically. The next day they are left feeling down, dejected, and alone.

Depression is having feelings of being down, useless, and disconnected. Anxiety is feelings of worry, anxiousness, and not coping.

Melancholy is a feeling of being both up and down at the same time, whereby you appear happy but feel like you are 'dying inside' (disguised).

In my experience, melancholy and depression may be present for many years but it is only when they **both** hit a low point, simultaneously, that affected persons feel and think that 'the world would be a better place without me'. Because of the nature of this mood condition, family and friends are left wondering why they couldn't or didn't see the terrible result (attempted suicide, suicide, self-mutilation) coming. The melancholic appeared happy (on the outside). It usually takes some major stress in their lives such as a relationship break-up, job loss, financial difficulties, issues with sexuality or justice, etc., to trigger the scenario of hitting this low point. However, melancholy was the underlying condition that created the opportunity to choose the option of death over life. Depression validated and intensified their disconnection and uselessness.

Melancholy has been described by some as being 'a reflection of death' and although we may have experienced feelings of 'it's not worth it all' at times, we cannot appreciate or understand how people with this condition think or feel. Some people say they have often felt like 'ending it all'. Teenagers sometimes use this ploy to get attention. Diligence is always the best ploy – by staying on guard. Only if they show melancholy and depression do I bring their family's attention to the risk of suicide and then start treating them immediately.

In my experience, this condition has a strong familial link. It doesn't affect everyone in the immediate family, but if you look deeply enough, there will be history of mental health disease, addiction issues, personality disorders, and suicide. Small children and even babies can show melancholic energy and tendency, for which we advise immediate treatment. Some parents and guardians ignore my findings, the need for treatment, and the follow-up care. Later they pay for their reluctance to believe that their family member could have such a condition. For some families, especially parents, the stigma attached is unbelievable. They personalise it, as if they have been bad parents – but melancholy does not relate to parenting or upbringing.

The origins of melancholy appear to have a spiritual/emotional connection, as if the melancholic has come into life with an escape hatch in case they choose not to be challenged by (or be accountable for) what they could learn from their experience in this lifetime. These people are not afraid of death and will often tell you they are fascinated by death, welcome death, and even fantasise about themselves dying. "When I die, people will realise how much they loved me; they'll miss me when I'm gone."

This condition only affects a minority of our population. Melancholic people often don't realise they are different to the majority and think that everyone in society has these feelings relating to life-versus-death choices. The older they get, the more aware they become that others don't experience these feelings.

Variable moods, ups and downs, the blues, the black dog, "the dark cloud that descends on my head", "get me out of here" (life), "the world is a better place without me", "I am not worthy of love", "I am a piece of cr*p", "I hate myself"; these are all examples of how these people describe their experience of being melancholic. The down moods may last from minutes, to days, to weeks and then upon snapping out of it, for no known reason, they cannot understand why or how they felt those horrible thoughts. Their lives are precarious as they don't know when these bad experiences are going to surface again.

These experiences usually surface early morning or when the person first wakes up. They know it is going to be a bad day. This makes sense as the person has been in a spiritual/emotional state when they are asleep. They may have been the life and soul of the party the previous night, but now they want to be left alone; they are non-sociable, withdrawn, aloof, angry, and aggressive. This behaviour can also be seen in children and teenagers – if so, it is important to get them assessed and treated.

My observation is that we have great results within two to three treatments. The patient and their families see changes because of treatment but also because of ownership by the patient, and enlightenment to the family.

Anxiety, depression, and melancholy often feed off one another and can be influential in displaying symptoms of any or all three conditions; however, if melancholy is present it is usually the driving force behind anxiety and/or depression. All three conditions can be mentally, emotionally, or physically driven and displayed but melancholy definitely has a strong hereditary/family connection that in adulthood spills over into the emotional/mental energies.

In severe cases, various forms of antidepressants are needed to balance body/mind chemistry while we attempt to balance the energies involved. Often a combination of medication and several treatments allow healing and stability of this challenging condition.

Following suicide (or attempted suicide, self-mutilation, etc.) parents or family members are often left wondering what they did wrong, or what happened to make their child take their own life. There is usually nothing they could have done that would have changed the situation other than if they were suspicious they should have sought help.

> *"When you reach that point of wanting to take your own life*
> *you are convinced the world is a better place without you.*
> *It is not about parents not loving enough."*
> (Bryan Hale)

Sean's Case History

Sean, a forty-seven-year old successful building-business owner consulted me to see if I could help him with the turmoil in his mind. He stated that he was a recovering alcoholic and drug addict, and with the regular support of 'AA' he had been sober for twenty years.

He ran a successful business and had a good relationship with his wife and three children, but stated, "Something is not right in my head."

Most days he was challenged by his past, but mentally he was able to cope due to the support systems he had acquired and chosen. However, he described how every few days he felt really down and didn't want to carry on living; he felt he was useless and that his life was meaningless. These feelings lasted anywhere from a few days to a week. He would snap out of it for a week or so and then it would return. There was always this feeling deep down that "life sucks", even though he knew that his life in other people's eyes was very successful and enviable.

He had sought my help through recommendations of patients at our office who had experienced similar feelings. He didn't want more drugs (medication) but wanted help to move on in life and "feel good" about himself and the great life he had created.

On examination, he showed cranial, neck, spinal, and pelvic problems due to previous traumas. His emotional and spiritual energies were very low. By contrast, his physical energy appeared to be quite high and his mental energy was extremely high. Depression, anxiety, and melancholy were all high too.

I explained to Sean that I suspected melancholy was his main issue. We agreed on a trial of three treatments which included structural work and the Hale Technique. On the third treatment, he walked in the door and said, "Mate, you have worked a miracle. I am a free man. Death is not following me around anymore!" On this visit, melancholy had just about gone from his energies.

He has steadily improved over six or seven treatments during the last two years. I now see him every four months for maintenance treatment. The second last time I treated Sean he asked me if I had heard of The Survivalist Movement? I answered in the negative. However, he must have been listening with openness to the conspiracy projections and was obviously affected by them as he showed up with an issue called Melancholic Depression; I balanced his energies again.

At the next treatment four months on he reported that within minutes of leaving the office the last time he had not experienced any more thoughts about such conspiracies and he was no longer interested in talking to anyone who was wanting to spread or talk about such negative stuff!!

I enjoy Sean's visits, especially when I advise him on what I have treated him for that day. He usually relates it back to some belly-laughingly funny story from his past.

Sean's history is: he started drinking alcohol on a social basis at age thirteen. By the time he was sixteen, he was frequently binge drinking and using recreational drugs daily. In his words, he was "zoned out on alcohol and pills daily" up to age twenty-two. At this time, he decided he needed to clean up his act as older men on the job started to question his competence as a builder. He continued to drink excessively and take recreational drugs from Friday night to Sunday night, then he'd turn up hungover to work on Monday and feel terrible for the next few days.

He loved music, and Keith Richards from The Rolling Stones was his hero. In 1995, he was very excited to be attending their New Zealand concert in Auckland; it was a dream come true. Full of alcohol and whatever other mind-altering substances he could procure, he saw his hero 'in person' for the first time, but because of the drug induced psychosis Sean had been in leading up to the event he actually saw Keith Richards as the Devil. Sean then reckoned that Keith Richards/the Devil started talking to him and told him that if he came backstage with the rest of the boys at the end of the concert they would initiate him into the world of Satan. Sean was horrified.

After having to be assisted home he finally sobered up four days later and vowed that he really had to do something about his addiction issues. Having tried many times before, this time it was for real, as in his words, "Mate, I'm not scared of dying, but gees, I'm bloody petrified of the Devil and going to hell!"

He finally went to 'rehab', sobered up, and has been clean since. In my practice, I have sent several 'out of control' addictive patients to Sean for a talk. I don't know what he says to them but every one of them has progressed very well since. Some people just have a gift and having travelled the journey they know the route and all the topography involved in reaching the desired destination. Sean is one of those special people.

One of his stories that appealed to me was: After two years of being sober, Sean's Mum and sister cornered him in the kitchen one day for a talk. They were concerned that he had lost most of his friends and also wondered when he was going to be able to drink alcohol again! It was at that moment that Sean realised that most people do not understand the serious nature of addiction issues in all its presentations. He asked his Mum and sister what friends they were talking about – "Jimmy the Junkie, Alex the Alkie, Dennis the Drunk, Bob the Boozer, Paul the Pisshead?"

Although medication is sometimes needed to assist and stabilise melancholic people it is both amazing and pleasing to treat them and observe such a quick change in their moods and resulting life. The various mind therapies and counselling, although helpful, in my experience do not appear to properly address this issue. Maintenance treatment with the Hale Technique is necessary on a four to six monthly basis to keep them stable, unless they experience some major stress, in any form, in between times.

Sean's case is very similar to many patients I treat presently. It is interesting that melancholic people's lives can be so agonising but when they decide to become real, accountable, and seek the appropriate treatment, they often become inspirational and dynamic leaders in society – the opposite to how they used to behave.

In my experience melancholy at varying levels affects approximately 20% of people I treat as patients. It seems quite likely that this condition could be one of the causes of criminal/addictive/rebellious behaviour seen in our society!!

CHAPTER 19

Stress

Stress is observed as being a major cause of illness in the body; however, it could more accurately be called the precipitator of underlying problems. Therefore, it can be likened to 'the straw that broke the camel's back'. The problems were pre-existing, but not observed; the stress brought these problems to the surface as symptoms indicating that the body was so overloaded with compensations that it could no longer adapt.

Other than accidents, the onset of almost every ill health or sickness experience is preceded either by the creation of stress or the relief of stress.

What is stress?

Our body and mind have to constantly adapt to our environment and challenges in life. Stress displays itself in symptoms and conditions that indicate to us that we are not adapting to and/or coping with those challenges. These challenges can be:

- **Physical** – accidents, injuries, sickness, not getting enough sleep or rest.
- **Chemical** – poor diet, sensitivities to medications, vaccinations, food/environmental allergies, hormonal imbalances, environmental pollutants such as pesticides, etc.
- **Thermal** – sudden changes in temperature, seasonal changes, inadequate heating, clothing, etc.
- **Mental** – most people identify with this type of stress as it is easy to recognise, if not by oneself then by those who are close to us in our lives.

Temporary and daily stresses, we generally adapt to easily enough, but it is the build-up of stressful situations that affect health by unbalancing body systems and energies.

In any stressful situation, the mental mind takes control by becoming over-energised. The energy is taken from the physical, emotional, and spiritual systems in order to gain this control.

Examples of how stress reveals health issues are:

- **Relaxation and stress relief. Physical symptoms caused by the *relief of stress* is the most common form of stress we see in our office. The patients say, "I cannot understand why I am sick, as my life has never been better and I've never felt so relaxed; stress levels in all aspects of my life are the lowest that I can remember. Life is great other than me being sick right now."**
- Before we go on holiday we work hard to get everything up to date before we leave. This requires a lot more energy, time, and effort, but because we are anticipating the holiday we consider it all worthwhile. The mental mind now takes up its superior position of being in control, anticipating anything that could go wrong while away on holiday – all possibilities are covered. We know we can control our thoughts and keep everything together – or so we think!

  When we finally go on holiday, the mental mind then relaxes – which exposes the under-energised physical, emotional, and spiritual energies. As they have been suppressed over a considerable period of time they now display their suppressed energies, presenting as symptoms of ill health and sickness. How many times have we looked forward to having a two-week holiday in the sun, relaxing, enjoying family and friends but instead we end up being sick the whole holiday? This experience is caused by relaxation of the mental energies, exposing the pre-existing suppressed energies caused by the mental mind's dominating control.

  This scenario can also be observed in experiences of prolonged stressful situations at home, work, study, completion of exams or projects where finally the task is completed and now it is time to relax. The mental mind relates to that but the other three energies may not!

- **Continued long-term stress.** As talked about in stress relief, the mental energies take control in any stress experience. However, unlike the above example, the mental mind can eventually become so overloaded that the person's coping mechanisms are at their limits. Another stress experience can tip the balance, resulting in a crash of all systems – now displaying symptoms of ill health and sickness. This scenario displays a far more serious picture as all systems have been pushed to their maximum and have now imploded, leaving quite a messy display of systems needing to be balanced and corrected.

    Generally, these people are very high-functioning individuals and have thrived by conquering many stressful situations encountered throughout their lifetime of challenges. What is hard for them to accept is that they are not 'bullet-proof' and like all other people they are human too. Their drive and coping mechanisms have in the past been exceptional but now that they have broken down, it is not always a quick and easy fix to bring them back to good health and high achievement again. Unlike relaxation of the mental mind, the continued stress experience has not only exposed their energy imbalances but has also exposed their issues with unresolved business in life, success, identity, purpose, goals, values, beliefs, etc.

    These issues have been the driving force behind their achievements thus far. The biggest challenge for them now is to accept and own their past behaviours and lifestyle, in the knowledge that they cannot go back to the old ways without experiencing the same results. Foremost, they need to accept their present health condition and position. Secondly, they need to understand how they got there and eventually, by finding self-forgiveness, they can now work smarter, not harder. Lifestyle changes can lead to decreased stress in life, less time at work, and more leisure time with family and friends.

Therefore, it can be stated: Ill health and sickness have a very strong association with not only body balance but also mind balance. Good health cannot be defined solely as being the lack of symptoms and disease.

CHAPTER 20

Fear of success

Fear is our most dominant emotion. When asked what their greatest fear is, patients usually respond with one of the following: failure, rejection, being alone, abandonment, death, life, and God[1].

From testing the body, by far the most common response is **fear of success**. Initially I couldn't understand this but after working with so many patients exhibiting this fear I have developed the understanding and techniques to deal with it.

> *"Have no fear of perfection: you will never reach it. Nothing in life is to be feared; it is only to be understood."*
> *(Marie Curie)*

People fear being themselves and instead identify with their job, their upbringing, and old teachings and beliefs. For example, if a patient has a fear of success they would test negative to "I am John Doe and I am a plumber, a father, and a husband" – with the self coming first. Meanwhile, they would test positive to "I am a plumber, a father and a husband, and my name is John Doe."

Fear needs a response immediately in a 'fight or flight' situation. **In order to give us more time and options when facing the challenge, we mentally turn fear into anxiety.**

---

1   *Wherever 'God' is mentioned the idea of a divine being or creator is meant (with respect to all beliefs).*

Both fear and anxiety flow between the emotional and mental sides of the mind. You feel anxious about being anxious. You think fearfully about feeling fear. Fear originates in our spiritual and emotional energies. In testing, you exhibit the fear of who you are and what your purpose is, leading into the two forms of purpose – materialistic and fulfilment. Once we try to control this energy by converting it to mental energy, we instinctively create fear of the unknown, of failure, rejection or judgment. "What if ... wait until ... too weird ... too weak ... where ... when ... why ... I don't want to."

We are by nature pack animals and it is more comfortable to stay with the tried and true, to be popular/well-liked and normal. If we step out, we believe that we may prejudice ourselves or be judged by others. We also fear that if we achieve success, somehow, we will have taken responsibility for other people and situations that presently seem out of our control. To have that extra burden is anxiety-provoking and unthinkable. However, that is just the mind making up more stories.

People say, "I don't know what I want to do in life." I say, "Yes you do, but so far you've only looked inside your mental mind. You haven't asked your heart because you're frightened of the power within."

"We are afraid of the enormity of the possible."
(Emile M. Cioran)

"He who is not courageous enough to take risks
will accomplish nothing in life."
(Mohammed Ali)

"Feel the fear and do it anyway."
(Susan Jeffers)

Not achieving your goals is not a mistake – it is a lesson. Writing goals down creates commitment, which leads to a greater chance of achieving short and long projections.

"What you get by achieving your goals is not as important
as what you become by achieving your goals."
(Henry David Thoreau)

"The bigger the challenge the greater the personal reward."
(Unknown)

"There is no challenge in easy."
(Maureen Rose)

"Adversity leads to opportunity."
(Unknown)

Experiencing Fear of Success

An example I tell patients is this: "Imagine yourself as a young child at the pool. A lot of friends are jumping from the high diving board. You very bravely climb up the ladder because you want to be accepted as part of the pack, but once you get to the top you look down and panic. When it is your turn you stand at the end of the board and fear goes through your body. To save face you have to jump, as the alternative is to go down the ladder in front of everybody. Within seconds you hit the water and you can't wait to try it again! You've now conquered your fear of that particular success."

The beginning of a journey starts with the first step. It is only the starting out that is fearful – what if you are successful? You have to believe that you will be assisted and guided by the Universe on your journey. Don't be afraid to speak and live your truth.

"Do what you feel in your heart to be right; for you will be criticised anyway."
(Eleanor Roosevelt)

Many patients have wanted new jobs that are pleasing and meaningful. Once they start working on the fear of success, the job finds them, not the other way around.

Adversity leads to opportunity. Be willing to dig deep and learn more. Overcoming this fear is not a quick fix but it is joyous for me to see that smile of freedom on people's faces when they conquer their fear of success. They now have freedom, self-worth, and own their life.

CHAPTER 21

Spiritual side

Often when spirituality is mentioned people either associate it with religious beliefs or turn off, dismissing the topic as being weird or spooky.

Initially I had trouble myself; now I don't let my mental mind get involved. Instead I have an open-minded approach without judgement. Acceptance that there is some higher energy in our universe is believable. People may have different ways of referring to such higher energy such as God[1], higher energy, or universal energy. When working with spiritual energy, we need to keep an open mind and remain light-hearted.

A few ways to identify your spirituality:

- A family with four children – living in the same household and having the same parents – are each unique, with different personalities, dreams, aspirations, and talents.
- You have five very close friends. Each of your friends has another five friends but you don't necessarily like all of them. Some you like or click with straight away – others you dislike or don't care for as soon as you meet them. Why is it that you don't like them and how do you know that you just don't? It is just one of those things that you know but can't explain!

---

1   *Wherever 'God' is mentioned the idea of a divine being or creator is meant (with respect to all beliefs).*

- You met and coupled up with your partner, wife or husband. Why? What made them more special than other prospective partners you had relationships with?
- Identical twins have different personalities and traits. You can attempt to explain this phenomenon (especially if you are over-analytical) but the reality is; **it just is**.

Your spiritual qualities reveal themselves in:

- Your **personality** – which is unique
- Your **instincts**
- Your **true purpose** – spiritual purpose – fulfilment
- Your **knowing** – the way you can just know something without knowing why or how you know it
- Your **sense of belonging** – your **identity**
- The relationship between **life as we experience it and the inevitability of death – death is the end of the present lifetime but is it the death of your spiritual lifetime?**
- The **unexplained connection you have to other things and other beings**
- Your **ability to be passionate and also to be 'in love' – especially with yourself**
- Your **connection to your dreams, whether positive or negative**
- How we **carry the blueprint plans for this lifetime – a blueprint plan is the master plan of what you have come here to learn and experience in this lifetime**.

> *"Nothing that God[2] ever made is the same thing to*
> *more than one person – that is natural."*
> *(Zora Neale Hurston)*

Your spirituality or soul is pure and often likened to **pure white light**. Energetic but not tangible.

---

2   *Wherever 'God' is mentioned the idea of a divine being or creator is meant (with respect to all beliefs).*

Through your blueprint plans you bring purpose into this life. The decision was made before entering this lifetime to experience your parents, your extended families, and your surroundings. You do this so that your spirituality or soul can experience and grow to a new level through the possibilities presented by the extremes of the mental mind.

The spiritual system is the messenger rather than the administrator and therefore carries no judgement or negativity. It is your mental mind that allows your limitless boundaries to achieve and learn, and it is your mental mind from which the spiritual (soul) gains knowledge. Eventually you die physically, mentally, and emotionally, hopefully having fulfilled your purpose by completing the lessons you came here to learn. Quite simply, you create a lifetime of stories, drama, and experiences as a 'student of life' who is in pursuit of mastering knowledge.

My beliefs/understanding from early childhood were very different to the formula I have listed below. This formula was developed from asking the following questions of hundreds of patients' bodies over the last thirty years; "Why are we here and what are we meant to be doing?" In other words, is there a meaning or purpose to life?

The formula

As a soul being we travel from one human life experience to another with a blueprint plan of what we want to learn and achieve in this lifetime.

We therefore choose our parents from our spiritual family in the location and surroundings in which we want to experience and learn.

Our challenges are created by the complex mixing of our Mum and Dad's families, hereditary strengths and weaknesses in personalities, characteristics, beliefs, attitudes, teachings, etc.

When this physical lifetime terminates and we 'wake up dead', our spiritual blueprint plan is presented to us for evaluation and analysis.

When we pass over, we analyse and judge ourselves on our performance regarding what we wanted to learn and achieve.

We're not judged by God[3], the Universe or others. The only judgement is from ourselves, which is the way it is meant to be. When we look at our

---

3   *Wherever 'God' is mentioned the idea of a divine being or creator is meant (with respect to all beliefs).*

world and surroundings we see both positive and negative situations and events happening for others. Unfortunately, we can only change our own environment (through making personal choices); we are limited in how much we can do to change outcomes for others. We can learn from our mistakes; **miss-takes** in any situation can be corrected by trying again, this time with knowledge. As they say in the movies, "**take two**". We don't learn from getting it right every time.

"I have not failed; I've just found 10,000 ways that don't work."
(Thomas Edison)

The difference between perfection and excellence is that perfection does not exist. The winner cannot continue to win every race. The place-getters may have performed their personal best times (that is excellence). However, if we make the same mistakes over and over again without learning and making different choices then we are stupid. As a practitioner, I see patients making the same stupid decisions repeatedly and then being bewildered by the consequences each time; however, because of their unwillingness to change, they continue to experience the same disastrous results. **Unfortunately, there's no treatment or remedy for stupidity!**

"Perfection is not attainable, but if we chase
perfection we can catch excellence."
(Vince Lombardi)

"Definition of insanity is doing the same thing over and
over again and expecting different results."
(Albert Einstein)

Through the journey that is life we are challenged by our spiritual system blueprint. Through the interconnection of our physical, emotional, and mental systems we make choices at each crossroads. Once we decide on a pathway, we are again challenged to choose another direction at the next crossroads, and so on, as we travel through life. The final stop is the physical end of this lifetime.

Until that time, we never stop learning and experiencing unless we decide to opt out temporarily, for a rest or permanently, when we refuse to learn anymore (lose the passion in life). It is our choice as we made the decision to come here in the first place. What are the ultimate goals for you in this chosen lifetime?

"Life itself is not difficult – living it is!"
(Maureen Rose)

The spiritual system is very pure and uncomplicated. It shows us what we're here to learn. Therefore, if we are, by choice, making poor decisions and behaving badly the spiritual system then 'opts out' by waving the white flag. (It literally goes into shutdown mode and surrenders; it only displays basic instincts.) This scenario is seen in cases of addictive, martyrish, and victimlike behaviour. It can also be seen in a moderate number of people who refuse to get out of the mental mind and experience their emotional/spiritual expression.

Various organisations, institutions, and individuals have used spirituality to gain law and order, power, and control over the masses or individuals. History displays the results of their actions and unfortunately this abuse of power continues to this day throughout society and the world; this is not the purpose of the spiritual system's existence.

God[4] is a word that to me suggests a higher or universal energy. It means different things to different people, and who has the right to judge others? From a treatment perspective, patients who are agnostic, atheistic, deeply religious, or even those who are conspiracists respond the same to treatment by balancing the four energies (PEMS[5]).

From many years of experimentation my experience has shown me that:

* No one can accurately predict the future.
* Past-life experiences have no relevance to healing or understanding in your present lifetime.

---

4 *Wherever 'God' is mentioned the idea of a divine being or creator is meant (with respect to all beliefs).*
5 *'PEMS' refers to the Physical, Emotional, Mental, and Spiritual energies.*

The past is useful in that learning to accept your past is good experience whilst on your journey. Accepting your past helps you to understand and eventually forgive.

Life would be easy if you could know what lies in the future and therefore be able to prepare for it. However, that would defeat the purpose of living your life!

The vast majority of souls that enter this world are good souls. They can become bad souls from continually making bad choices, leading to negative outcomes and behaviour. We have young souls, old souls, beautiful souls, sad souls, and complicated souls. Sometimes souls on the way to becoming bad souls have developed into **rejected** or **reticent** souls. I call this group **'R' Souls**.

Our most basic instinct is survival, which is intentionally positive – fight or flight. The mental mind can convert this experience into a negative experience. When we are in survival mode we expect a positive outcome – to survive. However, observation shows that often when people are in a comfort zone, thinking they have achieved their immediate goals, **they often turn survival into self-sabotage and self-destruction**.

The following case history may demonstrate this:

Nick's Case History

Nick, a thirty-seven-year-old salesman who was married with three young children had been a patient at the office for five years. His wife referred him for treatment of chronic lower back and neck problems sustained during his years of playing contact sports. His response to treatment was favourable and he expressed an interest in improving his health overall. In attempting this, his treatment was spasmodic and his behaviour was often unaccountable and victim-like (not turning up for appointments/not following treatment protocol).

I challenged him about his behaviour. He admitted that he was a binge drinker and an occasional recreational drug user. (Testing showed his 'habits' were low, demonstrating that although addiction was an issue he was not showing at a level that was needing specific treatment.) His relationship with his wife was struggling; his job and personal motivation were suffering too. We both agreed that he needed to do something to turn his life around. I advised him on a plan of attack to achieve this end and he was determined to follow this plan.

Six months later he came in for a tune-up/balance. He had lost ten kilos in weight, had stopped drinking alcohol, looked fit and healthy. He had a new job, which included a new car, and his relationship with his wife had markedly improved with couples counselling. He was a happy man, feeling loved and supported for the first time in his life!

I saw him again six months later. His fitness and life had improved further. It was now Christmastime and we discussed how his good choices had led to his present situation. All aspects of his life were positive and he was very proud of his success and achievements. I congratulated him and told him that I was proud to have been part of his achievements.

A month later I received an urgent call from Nick requesting to talk "in person", which we arranged. He told me that he had been feeling the best he had ever felt about himself and his life, so much so that he **wanted to celebrate his success** with a good friend by having one beer together at a local pub. The night ended up a long one. He says he does not remember much as he met up with some old mates and the rest is history.

The consequences were as follows. He lost his wife when she had to be treated for a sexually transmitted disease. He was charged with excess blood alcohol when driving and so he lost his licence and his job, probably his house and hard-earned assets too. No doubt also that his children will not be impressed as they grow older and learn about his behaviour!

I have seen many similar cases, maybe not as extreme as this one, but nevertheless demonstrating the same self-destructive behaviour. Peculiarly they still hold hope that they will be forgiven again and accepted back into their old life to be given a third or fourth chance!

Survival is our strongest instinct but its opposite side, self-destruction, often wins in the end, whether by choice or design! We all die eventually, but it is our choice as to the quality of life we choose to experience towards that end.

"People don't die, they just kill themselves!"
(Scott Walker – Founder of Neuro-Emotional Technique (NET))

Some treatments to demonstrate our work with the Spiritual System:

- **Nightmares or night terrors** – If you have witnessed this in children or adults, it is very confronting. The victims are not conscious and appear to be in a 'tranced but traumatised state'. Successful treatment is achieved in these cases by coordinating the spiritual reflexes and emotional reflexes with the five senses, which are smell, taste, hearing, sight, and touch.

- **Death issues** – When balancing the body, death shows up frequently when working with the spiritual system. **For some people, issues with death and dying are major. (There is one certainty in life: that is that one day we're all going to die.)**

    a) They can't cope with the fact that either they or someone else is going to die. Most people are not afraid of death itself, but they are fearful of how they are going to die with regards to the level of suffering and inconvenience this will cause others.

    b) They won't view or touch a dead person.

    c) They have a will to be dead themselves. (Statements like, "I would rather be dead than alive" vs "I would rather be alive than dead". This is a statement elicited in Melancholic or Depressed people, not at a physical or mental level, but at an emotional and spiritual level. They don't think (mental) or identify (physical) with "rather be dead" but they feel (emotional) and know (spiritual) that they would "rather be dead".

    NB. This phenomenon shows in any age group from babies to the elderly. When these people are confronted, most admit to this deep underlying feeling. However, loved ones around them would never know. This may explain behaviour that is devastating to family and friends when the patient has reacted to a major stress or upset in their life. Several treatments are required to treat this issue. Once balancing is completed the patient reports back that they no longer have those feelings and that death is no longer an issue for them. These patients are advised to receive maintenance treatment every four to six months as the shadow never completely disappears. After the initial treatments have helped them to achieve this state of being, they say that they actually thought that everyone experienced those feelings and thoughts.

We therefore cannot say that the mind is all-powerful and can overcome any situation, as if you are cast in that darker side of spirituality the emotional/mental expression is in the shadow of life, e.g. melancholy – rather than in the sunshine, which these patients automatically assume is how everyone is cast. We see it that way therefore we assume everyone is like us, but for some, they have come here to experience their shadow and learn by choices to accept help and treatment offered to them, and support by family/friends in this lifetime. In this lifetime, you may not see it, however when you wake up dead you will no doubt be faced with your options and the resulting choices that led to the final outcome.

- **Balancing the body's energies brings about burial of the past and creation of the new** – With most treatments, there is hopefully a realisation and acceptance of the patient's behaviour and belief system through balancing the PEMS[6] energies. At a spiritual level the body wants to visit death issues in order to begin a new era of personal development. It is as if we have to go back to darkness to restart the 'light phase'. This is similar to resetting the circuit breaker or the fuse in an electrical system of a house or rebooting your computer or cell phone.

When we are trying to understand life and death situations, we can liken it to the sun shining on a large glassy building, the sight of which offers visual pleasure. However, on the other side of the building a dark shadow is cast, which can be likened to death. They both exist at the same time, which is challenging for us to acknowledge as we are often 'in denial' about reality. Some people choose to only look at the light, some people choose to only look at the dark; people who are sensitive and anxious see both sides.

> *"Life would be tragic if it weren't funny."*
> *(Stephen Hawkins)*

Those who only see the light sometimes end up dealing with the consequences of not having considered what could happen in reality, during times of major adversity or in life-threatening situations. Therefore,

---

6   *'PEMS' refers to the Physical, Emotional, Mental, and Spiritual energies.*

they are unaccountable people as seen in cases of inadequate insurance cover, drink driving, not wearing a seatbelt, lack of vigilance with regards to their children's social media activity leading to serious repercussions, etc.

Those who only see the darkness are victim-like and cannot see any light at the end of the tunnel.

Often people dismiss anxiety/depression as being an excuse or weakness. One has to experience it to appreciate it.

Spiritual Expression is always challenging us!!

In September 2010, my learning experience was enhanced by experiencing a major earthquake, which caused structural damage to buildings and houses in my home town of Christchurch. Five months later in February 2011 another major quake occurred, with 185 lives lost plus further destruction and loss. The downtown and much of the business centre were destroyed and uninhabitable. Tens of thousands of houses had to be rebuilt or majorly repaired.

To this date there have been another 20,000 aftershocks and tremors, which appear spontaneously at any time of day and night. Stress has come from dealing with life amongst the chaos of uncertainty, but also from negotiating with insurance companies and local government agencies.

From experiencing these 'acts of God' (as insurance companies term these events), many adults and children present with major anxiety symptoms such as not being able to get off to sleep, not being able to stay asleep, experiencing panic attacks, etc. Most of these people have never experienced anxiety/depression symptoms before. **Interestingly, patients who have a history of anxiety or depression in the past seem to be 'in control' and have handled the earthquakes and aftershocks exceptionally well.**

Many of the earthquake-affected group have taken antidepressant medication and/or have received professional counselling, which has helped a lot, however many feel that "there is still something missing". Treatment with emphasis on emotional/spiritual balancing has brought about immediate and long-lasting relief that allows many of them to come off medication. The pattern shows that they have a **'fear of death' related to the safety of**

family and loved ones (external fear of death) as opposed to a fear of their own death (internal fear of death) as is/was common in the original anxiety/ depression group.

These experiences have presented a positive outcome for me as although I knew about the spiritual and inherited side of emotions, I had mainly treated patients with the internal fear of death in relation to spirituality. Patients have presented with emotional/mental crisis situations, but it wasn't until they presented with earthquake anxiety/depression en masse that I observed a pattern strongly linking the emotional/spiritual connection. This makes sense as our souls carry those lifetime experiences of persecution, famine, floods, earthquake, fire, etc. from other lifetimes (ancestral or genetic memory). These events have specifically surfaced old spiritual experiences into present day emotions of fear, anxiety, trust, sadness, persecution, etc.

There are always positives to be found in every negative situation. You just have to be open to opportunities presenting themselves to you!

What is the meaning of life? There is no meaning to life other than that we are here to learn, develop, and find our true purpose. Our soul or spiritual system is here to learn from our mental mind.

Our spirituality has no judgement, no analysis, no consequences, and no measured outcomes. It is merely the messenger carrying our blueprint and over the course of each human lifetime experience we have something new to learn. There is no hierarchical system either; you may be the president of the USA or the Pope in this lifetime. In the next lifetime, you may be a physically or intellectually disabled person, a prostitute on the streets of India, or a tribal person in Africa; it just depends on what you have decided to come here to learn. The spiritual side leads us to our challenges and obstacles in life. Our mental and emotional mind (through our values and principles) gives us choices, which are displayed in our behaviour.

To add to this colourful challenge we inherit various physical characteristics from our parents' DNA, plus we are majorly influenced by their teachings, feelings, beliefs, attitudes, intelligence, and behaviour. We have chosen our parents and hopefully one day we come to a point where we admire them for who they are and what they have done to nurture, love, support, and teach us.

As children, we all appear to have a common denominator in relationships with our parents. While we love our parents and maybe have grown to admire, respect, trust and like them, **we usually don't want to be *like* our parents – whether it be in personality or looks!**

A touch of understanding as to their intent and what was happening for them at the time can avert conflict and confrontation, which contributes to the healing process. If we look at ourselves and all other beings as 'individual souls', here to experience life for what we are here to learn, we should then be able to bridge the gap between genders, whether they are homosexual, heterosexual, bisexual, large, small, black, white, varying religions, different ethnic groups, etc.

If we are able to understand the intention of others (I suggest reversing the roles involved in the situation) we can stop 'reactionary behaviour'. Don't personalise the event, incident or situation. We tend to judge others and ourselves on outcomes and results rather than understanding the motive or intention of the person we are interacting with.

A common phenomenon that I have observed over the years with families is that the two family leaders (i.e. Mum and Dad) may have drifted apart due to them losing their spiritual connection. Mum and Dad got together by choosing one another as partners together in love. The offspring of this bond become the biggest challenge and job you will ever encounter in your life experience. They are your own flesh and blood and as family you will always love them, but **they are individual souls who chose you; not the other way around**. Herein lies a potential problem in relationships and family dynamics.

The order of priority in everyone's life should be:

First – oneself

Second – one's wife, husband or partner

Third – your children

Fourth – your immediate family

Fifth – your personal friends

Sixth – your job, profession or employment.

Seventh – your extended family and neighbours.

In relationship break-ups one partner can be left wondering what went wrong. For men, the answer is usually clear: "Once the children came along I was not important other than working to bring home money and provide for the family. My wife/partner became obsessed with the children so I found I had been replaced and superseded in the love stakes." This can even be true when the wife/partner also works outside the home. For women, the answer is also usually clear: "Once the children came along I was seen as just a Mum rather than a woman in her own right. I became someone who was just supposed to juggle everything and look after everyone else – and so my husband/partner stopped seeing ME." Children do require a lot of time and energy, especially when they are young – but don't lose sight of how that relationship started and what it created as a result. All relationships require constant attention, practice, and nourishment.

> *"We fall in love with individual souls, not with souls from a*
> *certain gender, race, or creed."*
> *(Maureen Rose)*

We as humans are not equal, nor do we have equal ability, insight, knowledge, intelligence or opportunity, but we do have the right to be *treated* equally.

In my observation over forty plus years in practice treating up to four generations of the same family, if they do not follow some personal development in learning to confront their challenges, they become their parents, both in behaviour and looks.

Many times, I have seen a son or daughter in the teenage years with stress symptoms related to dealing with the parent or parents. This creates in them a great number of physical symptoms from headaches, backaches, digestive upsets, etc. Often, they choose not to hear or follow through with treatment or what I have advised, but twenty years later they return with more serious problems and not only do they look exactly like their parents but they behave just like them too – the very behaviour that gave them so much grief and so many problems twenty years previously. When this is pointed out to them they acknowledge that this has happened and to make matters worse or comical (depending on how you want to view it), their own children are now challenging them in the same way that they challenged their parents!

Inherited family emotions have a major influence on outcomes in behaviour. Different generations of the same family show the same emotional characteristics that present the same symptoms, e.g. chronic allergies (food and environment), migraine syndromes, skin problems, digestive problems, back and neck pain, etc. Often the grandchild will tell me that I treated their grandmother for the same symptoms and that the emotional fault found was exactly the same. Interestingly I had no idea that they were related as being a typical man I would not have associated the two cases together.

In our office, we see families from grandparents to young babies. Often when checking the child, we come up with zero problems and no treatment needed. Through experience I ask Mum if I could quickly check her. Usually Mum explains that she does not have a problem, however more often than not we find issues spiritually between Mum and the child. Treatment of Mum results in Mum and baby/child feeling and functioning better and everyone is happy. In other cases, observation shows that the child may have problems that are treatable, however, if we are able to treat Mum first, the child's problems are not only less but they respond faster to treatment. Because of this, during a family consultation I always check Mum first and children later.

Another common phenomenon is that if Mum is present in the room when trying to examine and/or treat their child, we cannot find a treatable problem. When Mum leaves the room, the child now displays the need for treatment, which fits the presenting complaints and symptoms. A further bonus is that the child is better behaved and more compliant to instructions! Mum is the spiritual leader in most families. New life is conceived into Mum's womb and therefore becomes part of Mum's body and being, from time of conception.

In conclusion, there are very close connections spiritually/emotionally between parents and their children, especially with Mum. We don't fully understand these connections and how they all fit together, but I now accept that these connections are spiritually based.

The spiritual system is fascinating, exciting, and enlightening but we should be careful to concentrate only on the present and live in the now.

Honour, trust, and protect the energy of the spiritual system to help guide and challenge you in this personal life experience.

Healing Model

Learning and listening ❯ accepting ❯ understanding ❯ forgiveness ❯ healing

CHAPTER 22

Your life purpose

What am I meant to do?

Who am I meant to be?

What have I come here to do?

What is my identity?

What job suits me best?

What will make me happy?

These are all questions asked when looking for purpose in life. At some stage in our lives we all struggle with purpose and what our existence truly means.

As children, we are asked to dream about who or what we want to be. As young adults finishing our schooling we are faced with choosing a career pathway for the future. This is commonly our first real connection to purpose.

It is often when a midlife crisis challenges us, or we or someone we love faces a challenge that we are forced to confront the meaning of our lives.

These crossroads can take a lot of time and thought and sometimes it can be difficult to figure out where to start.

There are two types of purpose:

1. **Useful Purpose – Achievement of Success** (Status and Materialistic)

   This relates to your status in your occupation or job; however, it does extend into lifestyle, identity, assets, and social factors. Most people wrestle with materialistic identity. Pressure is imposed on us by ourselves and by others;

we worry about how we feel other people might perceive us – also known as the 'mirror image'. **How we see others see us is far more important to us than how we see ourselves.**

We live in a materialistic world. Our identity, motives, goals, ideas, reasoning, function, justification, and objectives are swayed by our job, car, money, house, clothes, image, friends, and colleagues.

Identity presents in many forms, e.g. gender, name, looks, health, financial wealth, success, education; usefulness, importance; belonging to family, group, profession, etc. Correction with treatment makes a big difference to finding identity, self-worth, and purpose.

My experience shows that when energies are unbalanced at an emotional/spiritual level then people with no identity in 'financial wealth' cannot achieve financial wealth, and women with no identity in 'gender' (as distinguished from sexuality) interestingly can show a history of chronic gynaecological and conception issues.

Owning and enjoying assets and comforts is good as they give us more choices for life, but drawing identity from those things does not give true or internal happiness. Rather they provide status, prestige, and position, and influence how we see other people see us.

I often ask patients what they think would make them happy. The answers often include things like winning Lotto; owning a home; meeting someone who loves them or makes them happy; being beautiful, slim, and fit; having a good job or being part of their/a family.

Having these things may create temporary happiness, but in reality, the happiness issue will reappear to challenge you again at some other stage if you have not acknowledged and dealt with what it is you really want in life. All of these things greatly influence our behaviours, values, and choices. We equate this type of purpose to **happiness** and **success in life**.

As humans, we see people with money and assets as being happy, which of course is not always true. Making money is often easier than holding on to it. If people with money are happy, it is because they are happy within themselves and through various choices they have made, such as less time working and more time having fun. Happiness can be facilitated by lifestyle.

Useful purpose relates to mental (thinking) happiness and it is therefore a **choice either to be happy or unhappy**. If you choose to be happy instead of unhappy, your changed attitudes and beliefs bring about different behaviour and outcomes because thought is creative. Success is achieved by fulfilling our goals (hopefully value-related).

2. **True Purpose** – Fulfilment in Life (Achievement, Accomplishment, Satisfaction).

   While useful purpose gives us identity, security, and comforts, true purpose is what we are aiming to achieve in life. Our true purpose relates to our creativity, usefulness, and personal satisfaction; this is how we achieve meaning to our existence in this lifetime. Through this we enhance our personal values and self-worth by living life for what pleases us (spins our wheels or turns our crank!). We do what we do for our own enjoyment, not according to how we think others or society may judge us.

> *"Tension is who you think you should be. Relaxation is who you are."*
> *(Chinese proverb)*

Personally, I struggled for years to find true purpose in my working life. Difficult as it was, I had to admit that what excited me about my work was that it gave me the opportunity to experiment on my patients, finding out what made them behave the way they do. Initially I was horrified that I was not more interested in trying to help them by relieving human suffering, but I had to admit that that idea came after experimentation, learning, analysing, and teaching others.

Owning this made me very satisfied and contented with myself as everyone ends up a winner. My learning enables my associates and myself to deliver more advanced treatments to patients, therefore delivering better results. My associates feel supported, our patients improve and refer others to our office for treatment, but most of all I feel fulfilled as my true purpose excites my existence.

You chose your blueprint for life, which leads to what you came here to do (true purpose), which in turn creates your lessons in life (challenges).

Some people put those challenges in the too-hard basket and give up. They may need more guidance and support to find their purpose.

Your true purpose will be clear to you once you can answer what it is you want to do to contribute to your world. We come into this world with nothing. We leave with nothing. What is it you want to achieve and/or contribute to your life's experience? You will never find the answer in your head (thinking), as the secret lies in your heart – as with fear of success.

> *"You cannot teach a man anything;*
> *you can only help him find it within himself."*
> *(Galileo Galilei)*

When you come to this position, you realise there is more to real happiness than what you have already achieved in life through just focusing on what others think. The secret is to be true to yourself and to dare to follow your dreams and realistic visions from deep down in your soul. Give yourself permission to be supported in your quest towards being someone unique and special. Honour your values. You will be supported towards finding true purpose.

If you have found your useful purpose, then true purpose is often easier to find.

Recognition of true purpose is more challenging than taking action to fulfil it. Peculiar as it may seem, family, close friends, and colleagues often see your true purpose long before you do. Sometimes it is feedback from others that helps you recognise what they see in you: strengths not yet recognised or owned by yourself. It is easy to deny who you are and be resistant to others' ideas and opinions.

The truth is, our loved ones are often right. As evidenced in confrontation – the vehement response usually indicates that a sensitive point has been revealed or that truth has been told! Opinions about true purpose often meet with a similar response. Our instincts and emotions create our useful purpose and our mental mind challenges them to create choices.

We ask questions like:

What about my security?

Where will I get the money?

How can I do that?

Who will support and help me?

What will people say or think about me?

This is often terrifying and we will be challenged by it. However, we only have to trust and be open to change while being accountable, caring, and realistic to ourselves and to others close to us.

"Life is either a daring adventure or nothing."
(Helen Keller)

As you read this, do you feel butterflies in your gut? If so, that is a good sign that **you have just been challenged!**

Are you truly and genuinely happy, or do you think you are happy? Happiness is an emotion rather than a thought so you should feel you are happy. True happiness relates to true purpose, not useful purpose.

Try this exercise:

- Look at your life backwards from your death to where you are now.
- If you were to die today, would you be satisfied or happy with what you have achieved or done in your life so far?
- Do you have unresolved issues with any member of your family, your friends, your work colleagues, or your neighbours?
- What do you want to do or achieve before you die? What are your aims and desires? If you don't have your goals written down, you are very unlikely to achieve them. Be realistic and sensible with these goals.
- What age are you going to die?
- What are you going to die from?

- Are you going to retire, or work until you die?
- Are you happy to go to a retirement home?
- What are your biggest fears confronting you presently?
  (Some examples are: worth, success, God[1], reality, being alone, abandoned, death, money, sex, knowledge, being loved or not loved, level of (dis)ability, health, etc.)

Answer these questions sincerely as they only matter to you.

Realistic Goals

If you do not have an intended plan, and/or goals in place, you will be blown around like a leaf in the wind, making no conscious choices in life. Making decisions gives energy to life as thought is creative and goals approached purposefully/seriously can be achieved.

Fate

Fate is the development of events outside a person's control, regarded as predetermined by a supernatural power, e.g. imagine a passenger in a car driving down the road. An opposing car goes out of control as it approaches. Unfortunately, all occupants in both vehicles are killed. Devastating. But these tragic events happen. Was it planned – who knows? Fate is fate over which we have no control.

On a positive note, there are lots of stories with great endings due to fate – many great relationships are created from fateful situations.

Karma

Karma, in my experience, is a theory not a reality. Do good people get rewarded and do bad people get punished?

> *"How people treat you is their karma; how you react is yours."*
> *(Wayne Dyer)*

---

1   *Wherever 'God' is mentioned the idea of a divine being or creator is meant (with respect to all beliefs).*

Personal Goals

In your goals, don't aim at materialistic things or assets. Work on success in family relationships, personal achievements, and harmony in your life.

Look at service to yourself and others, your personal health and fitness, travel and explore in your own area and district before going afar. Do the things you always wanted to do (have personal meaning or purpose to you). Start ticking them off as you go.

Interestingly enough, most do not cost a lot of money but do take effort, time, and planning. Maybe there is a reserve you drive past a lot and you often think to yourself that you must walk through there one day – just do it! Or there is a turnoff on the motorway that you pass a couple of times a year en route to somewhere else. The turnoff piques your curiosity but you never make the detour – make the time to just do it!

Write a eulogy for your own funeral. Mine is:

> *I die as a friend to my family and friends, without issues that*
> *I have created and continue to hang on to. I did my best*
> *with good intent and advice. I trust and pray that the world*
> *will be, in some way, a better place by my having been here.*

Is your true purpose in life to be a parent, grandparent, business owner, employer, employee, athlete, musician, artist, sculptor, teacher, inventor, or something else fulfilling to you?

It is the intent, the values, and the choices you make in performing these duties that create true purpose, not the fact of just doing it. There has to be some passion in performing and accomplishing that duty.

Questions you need to ask include:

- What is in it for me?
- What is in it for those I am serving?
- What am I learning and what am I achieving?

As stated previously, these questions can often be answered better by loved ones, family, and friends.

What pathway are you choosing to walk in life? The easy route, which poses few challenges, where everything is predictable and programmed, or the daring route, which challenges you to set goals and make decisions, allowing you to be an individual? Choosing this pathway leads to enthusiasm in your life.

"There is a certain enthusiasm in liberty, that makes human nature
rise above itself, in acts of bravery and heroism."
(Alexander Hamilton)

You have to make your choice on the route you take. The easy route poses large problems later in life when you are challenged and have little or no preparation or knowledge to cope or deal with adversity. The daring or testing route also poses challenges. However, because you have chosen to learn, your coping, and the outcomes are not only easier to deal with (but because of experience, learning, and knowledge), you may be able to see the positive possibilities or spin-offs.

Negative experiences and mistakes lead to opportunities for you to change – which means paving the way for a better future.

Nothing worth achieving is easy – approach it and challenge it. Curiously, once the process has begun it is no longer difficult or unachievable.

Some excuses are: "I don't know; It's too difficult; I'm too tired, too sore, feeling sick, washed out; I can't do it; I can't get out of bed." (If it was a matter of survival, such as the house was on fire, you wouldn't be thinking of your excuses!)

Can't means won't – set your mind to taking up the challenge. You may see only negatives, but once started you will find positives, just like getting out of bed in the morning when you don't feel like it. Just follow your plan and meet your challenges head-on and you will forget your ills and woes. Before long you will be having a good day and getting on with your life, fulfilling your goals, objectives, and dreams.

As Maureen Rose used to say:

"I owe, I owe; it's off to work I go!"

And

"Motivation is what gets you started. Habit is what keeps you going."
(Jim Ryun)

If you set your mind to fulfilling and achieving your goals, self-pity is only temporary. If your problems are permanent, seek professional help, and also honestly ask yourself:

"Do I want to get better?"

"Am I willing to listen, learn, accept help, follow the advice and treatment provided?"

"Have I honestly explored every avenue of treatment, both mainstream and alternative?"

These questions may seem heavy or philosophical, but are important to explore if you are not truly happy.

If you haven't satisfied and identified the purpose and reason for your existence, you are a burden to yourself and to all around you. Living with and spending time with an unhappy person is no fun, so you will find that others pull away, preferring to spend time and energy with progressive, interesting, motivated, and purposeful people, who are on a pathway of learning, and who are experiencing life.

Barriers to happiness

Excuses for not choosing happiness are:

• Some people turn their expectation of happiness into perfection.

  These people often have everything in a materialistic world, but because they lack purpose or fulfilment they escape into non-reality by wanting themselves to be perfect. As perfection does not exist, these people slip into deviant behaviour such as addiction, righteousness, and dismissiveness in an attempt to live in a perfect world. They blame everyone and everything in their lives for not providing them with a perfect world for them to live in. "I am the way I am because of ..."

- Other people get confused about where selfishness fits into their life.

a) To be **selfish** is to consider yourself and have your needs met first, while caring for and considering others second. This is a healthy choice and is the correct way of behaving and making decisions.

b) Some people live their lives putting others first at all times, and themselves second **(over-responsibility)**.

c) A step worse than over-responsibility is when they put others first and themselves last **(martyrdom)**. Neither b) nor c) are honourable, nor good for anyone involved.

People who live their lives carrying the load for others are always unhealthy physically, mentally, and emotionally. They have interpreted that because they give to others before themselves, somehow, they will be rewarded. Most friends and family see this clearly – the victims of these thought patterns don't and won't see it. They appear nice people to others but are self-pitying within their private lives. Behaving this way is an attempt to buy love, which rarely, if ever, works – as being a giver you attract people who are takers. They interpret that they are not appreciated for what they do for everyone. People close to them who try to help by making them aware of their behaviour usually experience an angry response.

d) Those who consider themselves first, last, and always (often at the expense of others), are **self-centred**. This is not good behaviour as they have no consideration for anyone but themselves – they lack feelings for others' needs, share nothing, arrogantly keep everything to themselves (this can be physically or verbally). **Unfortunately, this is what most people interpret as being 'selfish'.**

"To be selfish is good, as you put your needs first,
but have consideration and feeling for others second."
(Bryan Hale)

Emotions and their effect on physical health

Naturally our childhood behaviours are moulded by personality; gender; one's place in the family tree; ethnic, religious or family teachings; and also, beliefs and values. These influences are the basic foundations of our uniqueness as a person and how we see ourselves and our place in society. Understanding and accepting these basic foundations contributes to how we see ourselves, how others see us, and **how we think other people see us**. Ownership gives way to growth through different choices – forming new behaviours.

New behaviours lead to increased self-esteem, happiness, and hopefully acceptance by others. By achieving this acceptance, it is amazing what improvements in general health, well-being, and happiness result.

Mainstream and alternative health disciplines have the same basic objective of helping human suffering. Through belief and prejudice many practitioners spend a lot of time attacking other treatments – motivated by misunderstanding or competition – which means patients miss out. Temporary relief, in the form of pills or potions, make the most money. If patients heal and get better, they don't spend any more money. Therefore, most health organisations and pharmaceutical companies lobby third party payers – government, insurance – to pay the bills.

Statistically there appears to be very little difference in outcomes from the different forms of treatment, excluding crisis treatment. Although I value and admire counselling and mental therapy I find patients get stuck in the same old patterns. I myself have experienced more than twenty years of counselling and mental therapies with positive results only when challenged, and so in my practice, I refer to counsellors who actually challenge their clients. Without challenge, patients get stuck in their same old story, reinforcing their fear of success.

CHAPTER 23

Leadership

We play different roles in life according to the identities we assume in the various stations of our lives. Clarifying these identities helps patients to understand themselves and become 'in control' of all aspects of their lives.

Instinctively, we appear to have chosen before we enter this world whether we want to be:

- A born leader
- A facilitator (leader)
- A supporter (follower).

Born Leaders are born, not made, in the true sense. You can't be a facilitator or a follower and decide to become a born leader.

Facilitators are a type of leader. You may be a **supporter**, a **protégé** or a **victim**. However, with personal development and some goal setting, you may become a facilitator (leader).

Supporters are good people. They may not choose to stand in the frontline and make the decisions but rather follow the majority ruling. Protégés and victims, although different entities, have chosen to behave as such following personal challenges in life.

Born leaders may be: Teachers, visionaries, idealists, inventors, rebels, captains, healers, philosophers, tutors, gurus, and mentors.

To be a born leader poses great challenges in life. They often feel very alone, sad, fearful, and misunderstood. They tend to walk through life moving backwards, looking over their shoulder to check their intended direction. Moving along this way, they face the ground already covered, looking for facilitators and supporters who approve, trust, love, and forgive them as they move along their journey. They have to be reminded that a ship and an aeroplane steer from the rudder at the rear of the craft. Stop walking backwards looking for approval, love, and acceptance. Instead turn towards where you are going and if people want to follow and/or support you, they will. There will be fewer who do but the ones who choose to do so will usually be loyal and faithful.

A born leader wants to stand out or captain others. They are willing to go against the popular vote. They dislike rules or regulations and often have extreme views to the point of being rebellious. Facilitators are essential for born leaders to have around as they can cross the t's, dot the i's, make it all happen, clean up the loose ends, and bring it about harmoniously.

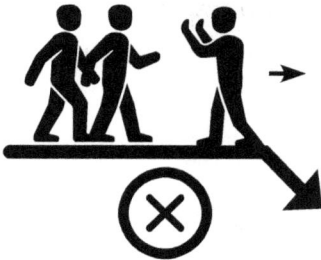

A LEADER WALKING BACKWARDS
SEEKING APPROVAL FROM BEHIND

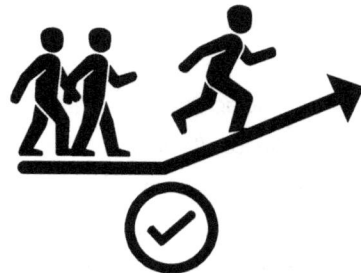

A SUCCESSFUL LEADER WALKING FORWARD
WITH THE TEAM FOLLWING IN SUPPORT

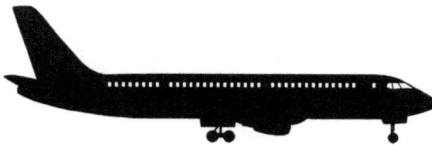

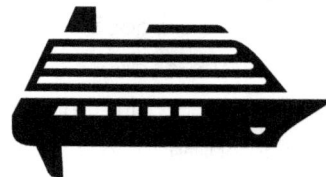

STEERING FROM THE RUDDER AT THE REAR

They often choose behaviours portraying martyrdom, betrayal, addiction, persecution, abuse, sadness, depression, and anxiety in response to being an outcast or different.

Instinctively, born leaders are great in certain areas of their lives but struggle (even to the point of being a victim) in other areas. For example, the person with a brilliant professional career, but who is disastrous in personal relationships and home life. On their journey through life they will regularly leave a trail of destruction or debris that needs to be cleared up by a facilitator or a supporter, as witnessed in most workable relationships. To further add to their despair, they never seem to see the trail they leave, and when it is brought to their attention take it as a personal affront or criticism. Born leaders need a lot of personal support, encouragement, and general maintenance to keep them focused and balanced, otherwise they may choose to opt out and become a recluse. Often, they are not good communicators and can't understand why others don't understand them or agree with their visions/insights. Frustration is often displayed as they see and know instinctively what others cannot even imagine could exist or happen.

Accepting and understanding that they are a born leader helps them own their behaviour patterns. This in turn gives the opportunity to change how they act/react, heal their relationships, and forgive themselves for having chosen a born leadership identity in this life.

Facilitators may be: Teachers, team leaders, managers, accountants, lawyers, and police.

A facilitator is a type of leader as they coordinate, promote, help, make things easy, and pave the way for groups to agree on a common goal, purpose or pathway to bring about a result or direction. Therefore, they can be group/team leaders, sub leaders, facilitators of ideas and actions. Negotiation is their strongest ability and unlike born leaders they can see others' views.

They are usually forgiving, gracious, realistic, accommodating, helpful, and purposeful. Although they are not looking for supporters, they tend to spend more time and energy on those who don't agree with the philosophy, direction, and purpose of their group, so like leaders, they can be challenged by martyrdom, betrayal, addiction, persecution, abuse, sadness, depression, and anxiety. There are varying levels of facilitation – relating to ability, communication, and knowing.

Every leader needs (and looks good) if they have a good facilitator in their team. Behind every great man/woman (born leader) there is an even greater facilitator. Most people would like acknowledgement of this identity as we seem to aspire to be leaders so as not to be labelled a follower (supporter). Facilitators are usually balanced leaders who may need encouragement and support, but don't have the highs and lows of born leaders. They live with more reality.

Protégés: This identity is a difficult place to be in as these people need a lot of encouragement and support to move through this transitional stage (transformation) from having been a supporter or a victim to being independent and self-reliant.

Once this is achieved, they can gain the confidence to become a facilitator/leader. The dream, the will, and eventually the choice, are all essential as one can become the dream if one believes and wants it enough. This applies to any level of identity whether you live in it or outside of it. As in sport, the earlier you make the decision, practise and perfect your work/skill, the quicker and easier the transition and transformation. Age is not a barrier, just a state of mind when you are dealing with behaviour that is determined and monitored by the mind.

Supporter: A supporter is a fan, admirer, believer, pupil, representative, attendant, and assistant. These people are not weak or powerless, but instead are very passionate and motivated with a strong sense of belonging. They are often highly principled with good values and high ideals, which can lead to either good or bad behaviour, or a combination of both, depending on the situation they are in. Groups or teams with rules and regulations suit them best.

They are strong on loyalty, purpose, principles, philosophies, beliefs, agendas, and their group identity. As a result, they can be righteous, sensitive, fearful, non-trusting, persecuted, sad, angry, guilty, and easily betrayed. Structure, familiarity, routines, and guidelines favour supporters as they like to know where they stand, what is expected of them, their position at work/life/home and where in the group they fit regarding power and responsibility. Their stresses are basic instinctive ones as they choose to fit into a structure or organisation in which everyone shares the burdens so as to have a sense of identity and belonging.

Victim: Victimhood is a choice of identity in which the person has given away their power due to being one of the three aforementioned identities. They are a sufferer, injured party, scapegoat or prey to another person, a situation or circumstance, resulting in them choosing to be victimised, persecuted or bullied. It develops into a way of being in which their behaviour is compromising and challenging to everyone in their life.

They have no power, cannot make decisions or stand up for themselves, which makes them unreliable, untrustworthy, unaccountable, indecisive, and the list goes on. Confrontation ends in them either being totally passive, subservient, running away, hiding, making excuses or becoming angry, aggressive, self-pitying, vengeful, or blaming others ('Poor me' syndrome).

"You are running out of people who will listen to you or believe you."
(In Maureen's words)

Bullying

Being bullied is a symptom of victimhood. The only way you can stop bullying is to stop the victim being a victim: bullying relates to over-responsibility. Once a bully finds a willing victim, the relationship is symbiotic. Victims either attract bullies or through their behaviour make others close to them behave like bullies (actively or passively). Bullies victimise others in order to exert power and maintain control. A seldom acknowledged dimension to bullying is when the bully bullies their victim whilst subconsciously thinking, "If I bully you into being my victim, I can look after you, i.e. put you first in my life and protect you. In return, you will look after me because you owe me for my protection. Together we are stronger as a unit than either of us having to stand up for ourselves."

The bully does not comprehend that their 'controlling by force' behaviour is unhealthy for both parties. Conversely, as victims have given up their power and control their vulnerability is obvious to others, who are emotionally removed and looking in at the situation from afar. Bullies have a strong element of victimhood. They most often graduated from a victim to a bully because of size and age. Most often bullies have a history of being bullied themselves.

Our behaviour displays different types of identity, depending on what part of life we are experiencing challenges in. You may be a facilitator but live certain areas of your life as a victim. However, we get stuck if we try to live our lives applying different identities to different areas of our lives. You are who you have chosen at some time to be – a born leader, a facilitator, a supporter, and later in life perhaps a victim – therefore you should be living that role in all aspects of your life.

Questions we practitioners ask the patient's body are:
- Am I a born leader? A facilitator? A supporter? A victim?
- I live my life as a ...
- I am a ... at home in my immediate family.
- I am a ... in my extended family.
- I am a ... in my work, my job, my profession, my school, my learning institution.
- I am a ... in my personal relationships with partner, friends, work colleagues.

If they don't get the same answer to all six questions, then corrective treatment is necessary. The treatment changes the energy. The patient is now aware so they can choose to use that energy to effect healing.

Low self-esteem, anxiety, confusion, and frustration are often replaced by acceptance and understanding when these areas are balanced. You may be a born leader but live most of your life as a victim, or you may be a supporter and live your life partly as a leader and partly as a victim. Identifying and balancing the energy helps patients to understand why they have been behaving in a different way according to their environment at the time.

Whatever identity you have chosen or are living, the big question you have to ask yourself is, "What is in this for me?" In other words, what do you get out of being or behaving this way? Do you behave this way in expectation of some reward or because of your values and principles?

If you do not have any expectation of outcome for your contribution, ideas, and input, you are contributing freely and unconditionally and therefore eliminating judgement, guilt, fear, hope, approval, etc. – not so much from others but more for yourself.

CHAPTER 24

Forgiveness

Forgiveness is the most powerful contributor to true healing, but it is the most difficult process to achieve. Self-forgiveness is the key to starting this process.

You have reached a state of forgiveness when you feel able to relinquish your desire to punish yourself or others who have wronged you. It is rewarding to be able to move on from that desire to 'get even' and to feel in control of how you 'give' (conditionally or unconditionally) in the future.

Through 'questioning' patients' bodies I have developed an insight into how to address the ownership of forgiveness. Unconditional forgiveness (to give without expectation of a reward or return) is possible but rare in humans. Even dogs (who give unconditional love to their masters) are guarded when it comes to forgiveness. Conditional forgiveness is the usual state I see in people. Despite some people claiming that they do things to make others happy, there are conditions; this normally involves the expectation of something in return, even if that something is only love and approval. Most would rather give than receive. Receiving creates the feeling that you are indebted to the giver and that you need to give in return. Giving creates self-power. Giving the way you have in the past may not have worked in a healthy way for you and so may have affected your self-esteem and worth. If this is the case, you need to learn from experience and change the way you give in the future to both;

- yourself and
- to the person/situation you had that experience with.

To change the way you give, you need to work through the process of understanding yourself and your relationships with people, and how you react in situations you are faced with. You should not continue to give energy, time, and meaning to relationships, people, and situations if they cause you to feel compromised and/or out of control.

Additionally, do not confuse being 'in control' with 'controlling' other people or situations

- To be **in control** is **empowering**
- To be **controlling** is **disempowering** for all parties involved.

Self-forgiveness

To reach a state of forgiveness you need to understand the reasons you might continue to give of yourself to people/situations. The most powerful act of forgiveness is self-forgiveness.

In past relationships or situations, you may see that you acted inappropriately, maybe from lack of knowledge or from trying to gain some sort of justice or recognition. Accepting, owning, and understanding why you behaved as you did can lead to forgiving yourself for the creation of your dysfunctional relationships.

I spoke to parents regarding one of their sons (in a family of four children) who was difficult and challenging to everybody during his teenage years. The parents tried their best but that one child's personality meant that he was more demanding and difficult, required more energy, resources, and time than the other three children put together.

For that particular child, accepting **ownership** of his attitudes, behaviour, and also of his comments such as "it's not fair, they get more than me, they had more opportunity, money, time spent on them", etc., helped him to understand why he was treated the way he was by the others.

Ownership, along with giving ourselves permission to leave it all in the past (as that is where it belongs) creates new energy towards self-forgiveness, leading to forgiveness *by* others. By achieving this milestone, forgiveness *of* others is automatic, which will be reflected in behaviour by all parties involved.

Self-forgiveness removes you from the victim role and directs energy towards forgiving others, rather than giving energy to relationships and situations that disempower you. By holding on to the past, you may be hoping for either an answer or a change in the person or situation that caused it. The energy remains the same. Many times, patients just want the offending party to see the error of their ways. That rarely happens because the offending party usually does not recognise that there is a problem with their own behaviour or that there is a need to apologise. There is no winner when each party feels the fault is with the other side. By admitting and owning your past behaviour, the energy is moved towards healing yourself, which in the end is all that matters. You cannot heal or control what others do or think, but you can choose to end your victimhood. Empowering yourself through ownership puts you 'in control' of any situation relating to forgiveness issues of self or others.

There is often a pattern where individuals are attracted to certain personality types and get involved in personal relationships despite knowing how this person has behaved in the past. If you experience this then you must learn to forgive yourself for your 'miss-take' and learn to avoid that personality type in the future.

"What can you expect from a pig but a grunt."
(Old proverb meaning why would you be surprised by poor
behaviour from someone you know to be rude, etc.?)
(In Maureen's words)

Perceived abuse by parents is a common issue we hear about in practice. This may take the form of physical abuse or mental abuse by using persecution, abandonment or betrayal. Move to acceptance by believing that your parents were doing their best with the knowledge and skills they had at the time and always remind yourself that it is impossible to change the past. Ownership and acceptance of your behaviour towards your parents during your childhood promotes understanding as to why they reacted to you in the way they did. Reverse the roles and try to see your relationship from their perspective. Did your parents disciplining and raising of you differ from how they treated other siblings in your family? The usual answer is "yes, they treated me differently", however other siblings and parents explain that it was because the said plaintiff behaved in a challenging manner that required impromptu responses in order to cope with the situation in hand. Many times, I have observed the victim feeling abused or persecuted when in fact the parents were putting safety, security, and common sense before the unreasonable requests or demands being presented by an uncompromising child, teenager or adolescent.

Abusers, persecutors, abandoners, and betrayers are often mentally ill. They have no excuse for their actions and there is usually no justice or reconciliation either. There is a way to release yourself from being their victim by attempting to understand them and yourself in the relationship that developed. The fact is, in consenting relationships there are always two sides to every story. Ownership of your behaviour initiates the process of forgiveness (which is not a quick fix). Victims may need counselling and guidance to get them started on a journey of acceptance and understanding.

To truly heal the past (as it is the past, not the present nor the future) is to come to a place where you thank the perpetrator for the experience. They were your teacher and you were their unintentional pupil. You were affected by their behaviour while they possibly did not (and to this day still may not) understand why you have these issues!

The probability is that they will never 'get it' but you can heal through forgiving yourself for the experience of learning. Hopefully, through your learning, you will break the cycle and enable your own family to have a better experience than you did. Often those who choose to heal have not recreated any of the situations they personally experienced with anyone else in their family or life. The chance for these people to help others by supporting and setting an example to others who are trapped where *they* used to be enables them to heal further themselves.

Many patients have difficulty in accepting 'forgiveness of others' as a possibility because they feel an obligation to change the offending party by having them see what trauma they caused in their life. Somehow, even if the person has passed away, the victim would like them to know how they have suffered. "There must be some justice in life" is often how they feel. However, unfortunately this is usually not the case.

Hard as it may seem, forgiveness is possible and wonderful healing is created by surrendering the energy you once gave to that relationship or situation.

"The emotion that can break your heart is sometimes
the very one that heals it."
(Nicholas Sparks)

As a child or adolescent, you may not have had the resources, protection, support or opportunity to avoid becoming a victim of the given situation but as you grow older you can move on. Some of the most inspirational people I have met have been through major abuse situations in their childhood, but after various experiences of desperation later in life have agreed to accept help, advice, and treatment to arrive at a place of being truly awesome, inspirational leaders and teachers in our society. Sadly, the opposite sometimes applies to privileged people who have not embraced their opportunities.

Forgiveness and abuse are similar in that, each time you face the issues and remain in control, the more the scars of the wounds fade. I have seen many cases where patients are working on their issues of abuse, betrayal, persecution, and abandonment up to thirty years later, still looking for resolution.

"If you don't like the hole you are in – stop digging and looking
for answers – the hole is only getting deeper!"
(Unknown)

There is no resolution, apology or justification for what you experienced personally. Leave it in the past. Forgive and leave it where it was. It is no longer affecting you, unless you keep giving it energy in your present life. Learn to let go and forgive yourself for the lessons learned but never forget the wonderful opportunity you were given to change your personal world. You have managed to turn things around so that your world is a better place; you can now experience love, and both you and your family will benefit from that.

Forgive, but never forget. Many do the opposite, trying to forget but not forgive. This leads to ill health and bad behaviour. Often the person thinks they have forgiven, but through testing we see that the body disagrees.

This must be done actively, not passively nor dismissively. You need to point out to the person you are confronting (disagreement) that you are unwilling to proceed to conflict (willing to fight) stage. They are entitled to their viewpoint, as you too are entitled to yours. Refusing to enter into confrontation or else dismissively walking away in the first instant is disrespectful and tantamount to inviting conflict.

By changing the way you behave, the other party is forced to change their behaviour if they want to engage you. Follow your values, not your beliefs.

Counselling by a professional therapist is the best way forward if mutual respect and honour cannot be achieved.

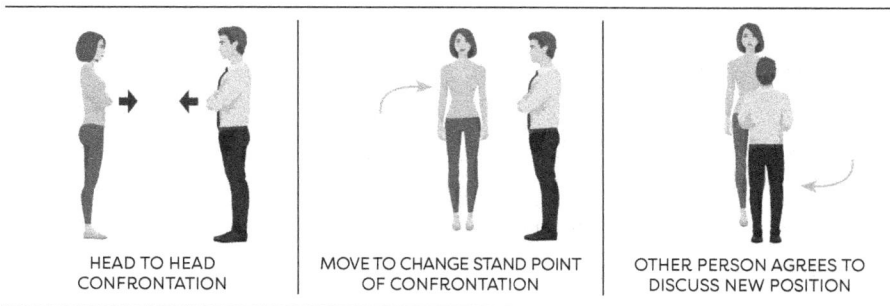

HEAD TO HEAD CONFRONTATION | MOVE TO CHANGE STAND POINT OF CONFRONTATION | OTHER PERSON AGREES TO DISCUSS NEW POSITION

From observation of marriage and relationship break-ups, it is so often the case that the unhappy partner who initiated the break-up is still having the same problems for years later. The other party, while hurting initially, has had the opportunity to work through a grieving process, learned to forgive, and moved on, usually finding a great new relationship within a few years. The majority will say that they are glad that the break-up occurred and that their ex-partner did them the biggest favour ever as they have never been happier!

Repeated criticism of, and unhappiness with others, is usually indicative that the said person is looking in the mirror, projecting their own issues onto others.

Forgiveness is a process. Once you start owning the concept of how you and others have behaved you start to forgive and heal many areas and relationships in your life. Harbouring grudges leads to hidden negative/hostile thoughts. Ill health and disease develop because energy is out of balance. **Our most powerful instinct, survival, switches to self-destruct mode.**

By forgiving you create the opportunity to learn, heal, and teach others; there is no better reward or contribution to society.

Forgiveness leads to peacefulness. Once you start achieving and experiencing peacefulness you have created an unstoppable love and passion for yourself and your life.

Peacefulness is a state of being in control of both the emotional and mental mind. Good people become great people when they achieve this.

Over the years, I have worked with people who have chronic allergy type symptoms such as hay fever, skin rashes, gut problems, headaches, and chronic viral infections.

Many of the younger people who are troubled by these symptoms are delighted when their symptoms spontaneously disappear while they are away from home travelling or working overseas. However, when they return to their family and home environment, the symptoms return with vengeance. They explain that the symptoms returned when they were close to landing back in New Zealand and that it must be the air in New Zealand containing antigens and pollens, etc., causing their allergy/health problems to return! This rationale does not make sense especially since the air on the plane is not New Zealand air! Testing often shows that they have not addressed past issues relating to forgiveness with family and/or friends. Busy overseas, they put the issues to the back of their mind but coming home means having to face them again. These patients need to urgently address these issues and as their practitioner I can usually tell them who and what the issue relates to. Acceptance, understanding, and eventually willingness to work with the process are all necessary to balance the energy and help the body heal.

The three the most common experiences for patients where they will need to master forgiveness are:

1. **Break-up of marriage or a long-term relationship.**

   Typically, it takes at least two years for the grieving party to come to terms with their traumatic experience, however if they can achieve forgiveness, they become a stronger and healthier person overall. Initially they maintain they have done nothing wrong so believe that they do not need to practice self-forgiveness as the other party is at fault. It must be pointed out to them that **they were responsible for contributing 50% of growth and commitment to their previous relationship**. Did they put in energy and time, agree to mediation or counselling, communicate, listen, and try to improve any aspect of the relationship or did they take the partner or spouse for granted?

Ownership and acceptance of their behaviour in the relationship will ideally promote some understanding as to why they have ended up being the victim. If they can reach a point of acknowledging how they got to where they presently are then self-forgiveness is achievable. Self-pity and laying the blame on others further complicates troubled relationships, plus creates communication issues with family and friends.

Once they choose to move on, self-forgiveness eventually leads to forgiveness of the offending party. In doing so, it is usually not possible to re-establish the relationship in any way like it was, but it is possible to have civilised encounters especially if children are involved. Problems only arise if both parties agree to continue a relationship of conflict rather than allowing forgiveness to prevail by learning from the mistakes of both parties in their past.

2. **Fallouts and disagreements within families.**

There are very few families who do not experience conflict between their members, whether they be parents, children, in-laws or extended family. Because this group often comprises of a large group of people, statistically it is more likely that there is a wide variety of dysfunctional behaviours amongst its members. In my opinion, family equates to dysfunction as we have chosen our families to learn from in this lifetime.

Parenting is the most difficult job that you can ever undertake. Children are uniquely different individuals and the way parents have disciplined them or raised them may not be individually received in the spirit that was intended or given. I hear many parents blame themselves for how the children ended up as adults. In simple terms, you raised them to the best of your ability – nurturing, teaching, and guiding them in values with what you knew best at that time. It is up to them what they do with those gifts. Move on by not giving the relationship any more energy other than acknowledgement. Love them as your child but respect, trust, and liking must be earned. Leave it there, move on but most of all forgive yourself, as if you had your time raising them again, would you have done it any differently unless you had the knowledge you have now?

The child-to-parent relationship is more difficult as there is often a sense of entitlement present, along with issues of approval and subservience that become involved in characteristic behaviour of sons and daughters towards parents. Ownership of these issues is essential, as well as asking questions about how they behaved as a child in relation to their expectations of how they assumed their parents should have treated them. Was there any consideration of what was happening in their parents' lives regarding relationships, finances, security, and other family issues or was it all about them in a self-centred, self-pitying mode?

Often when I question children about their parents and/or other family members, there is a clear picture of major depression/anxiety, post-natal depression, post-traumatic stress syndromes, etc. In the past, there were not as effective medications, counsellors or help for such problems as there is now, let alone acknowledgement of or acceptance by society in general, that these issues could even exist.

Communication is the best healer of any confrontation and/or conflict. Listening to others and trying to understand them; these are the strongest attributes of communication.

3. **Loss of a loved one by accident or death.**

Fate is unfortunately something that we cannot explain. When a tragedy occurs in our life we tend to blame ourselves, others, God[1] or the Universe, to try and make sense of why and how it happened. We say there must be something we could have done or said that may have saved the situation or altered the outcome. We also sometimes grieve because we know that we should have shared our love with them over the years but, unfortunately, it went unsaid.

---

1   *Wherever 'God' is mentioned the idea of a divine being or creator is meant (with respect to all beliefs).*

Nothing is going to bring them back or recreate the same relationship we had with them when they were alive. Some comfort is gained by imagining them no longer suffering or in pain, having moved on from their physical world to a better place.

This experience is far more traumatic for us because there was no choice (apart from suicide – another issue) by the deceased to leave us and therefore forgiving them for what has happened between us is not difficult. Forgiving ourselves for not fulfilling wishes such as "we could have, should have, would have" as expressions of love, is possible.

As with abuse and abandonment issues the scars of this experience often run deep, but if we can forgive ourselves and stop trying to blame and find reasons for the loss, we can achieve self-forgiveness and acceptance that we did not and could not have done anything better for a situation or event that was totally out of our control. Maybe in another place and time we may understand. The biggest realisation is, there is only one person still hurting and that is the person who needs to self-forgive.

All behaviours are repetitive unless they are either challenged to change or if we reach out for forgiveness through accepting and understanding other people's perspective and experiences. Acknowledgement that there is an issue to be addressed is a major step in ownership. Understanding is then only a short step away.

Hopefully, by understanding the process set out above, it may help you, the reader, to achieve forgiveness of yourself first and others later.

Lucy's Case History

Lucy, a twenty-six-year-old student consulted me for relief of migraine headaches, sore throats, and abdominal pains. All the symptoms started approximately fifteen years ago. Over the last year, she had been experiencing daily headaches, mouth ulcers, and also feeling bloated and nauseated. She had been taking medication for asthma since childhood, was taking the contraceptive pill, and in the past few years had experienced frequent episodes of vaginal thrush. She complained as well that her energy was low and that she had trouble getting to sleep and staying asleep.

Both her mother and brother had always experienced frequent migraines.

Examination and evaluation showed a hormonal imbalance, structural problems with her pelvis and skull plus major stress-related emotional/mental imbalance.

Lucy's case was difficult because of the emotional/mental overlay to her symptoms; however, she was treated six to eight times over the next two years. Her headache issues, sore throats, abdominal pains, mouth ulcers, and thrush responded favourably.

Over the next twenty years she consulted me two to three times per year for stress relief relating to issues with her family, as they were hard-working farming folk while she was very arty, spending most of her time singing, painting, and acting. During those years, she gave birth to two wonderful children. Approximately seven years after the youngest child was born she was delighted to be pregnant again with a third child.

Unfortunately, during the eighth month of the pregnancy the baby's heart stopped and so the infant passed away in utero. Lucy was totally devastated and it took her a full two years to recover enough that she could function normally again. It was as if her whole world had collapsed in on her.

During this time and for the subsequent seven years I rarely saw Lucy as a patient. Then three years ago, in desperation, she consulted me again seeking help for uncontrollable anger, anxiety, depression, and a multitude of physical symptoms.

Again, I treated her with some positive results, however her emotional/mental health was not stabilising and improving. I confronted her about her ongoing victimhood and lack of forgiveness towards her family as that was what her body was indicating from my testing/findings. As expected, World War III erupted, as it usually does in these situations where I choose to challenge patients on their behaviour. Naturally she was extremely upset with me and told me so. As I explained to her I was only the messenger and so was just delivering the message her body was telling me. She texted me to tell me that she was so disappointed that we had shared a doctor-patient relationship over twenty years. I communicated back to her that I couldn't see her go through the years ahead suffering mentally and physically. As a practitioner, I would feel a fraud not telling a patient the real truth about a condition I see as being a noose around their neck presently, and also going forward.

She returned for treatment a week later after thinking about what was said. Through a process of me challenging her I explained to her the effects of her behaviour on her family and friends. At this time, she was still not convinced but agreed that she would go away and think about it.

A month later she consulted me again and I could not believe the person walking through the door was the Lucy I used to know. She said she went home and thought about it, talked to her husband and some friends, who all agreed with my assessment of her behaviour towards her family over the years. They all agreed with me that her family was not even aware that there was an issue as the family's interpretation was that Lucy was one of those artistic people who are a bit strange, totally out of control, always looking for attention and money.

Lucy began to own her behaviour and her attitude towards the family, realising that she was the only loser in the family circle. This helped her to understand that her family were not capable of recognising and appreciating who Lucy was on any kind of emotional or spiritual level.

She immediately stopped trying to change them and get them to see her viewpoint and her achievements in life. She also stopped looking for an explanation or an apology.

In her words: "They will never get me and who I am!"

Over the next twelve to eighteen months she became progressively stable, happy, and a lot healthier, but most of all she is free and at peace with herself. It will take time to reach a place where she is at peace with respect to her relationship with her family, but already she wonders why it took her so long – with all that wasted time and bad energy. Naturally her relationship with them will never be the same, but they will probably all go to their grave wondering what happened to Lucy from the year she reached out and achieved forgiveness of herself and them.

Lucy now has the power and says she can't stop grinning when someone mentions her family.

What great teachers she chose!

CHAPTER 25

In conclusion
(as a practitioner)

I hope that when reading this book, you have come to a conclusion that good health involves a lot more than having a healthy diet, keeping fit through regular physical exercise, taking prescribed medications, supplementing your diet with nutritional products, and avoiding stressful situations.

One's hereditary and genetic factors along with education and environmental, ethnic, and religious teachings and beliefs are all contributing factors towards how we choose to behave and experience our lives.

The mind, comprising its emotional and mental components, is the controller of how we display behaviour and choose life's challenges. Personal health can be described as a reflection of how our physical body acts and reacts to our total environment, which can be another way of interpreting stress.

Stress is not the sole major cause of disease/illness but observation shows it is a major contributing factor in surfacing underlying, pre-existing health conditions, e.g. a person may have cholesterol issues in their body. Experiencing high stress or relief of stress may surface this problem by them experiencing a heart attack or stroke. The problem was pre-existing; experience of stress surfaced the resulting condition.

As discussed in this book, emotional/mental energy imbalance creates physical energy imbalance, which over a period of time displays in the body as symptoms. And with any health condition, no matter what the cause, the emotional/mental energies are affected merely by the fact that the patient has pain and is not feeling well (general malaise).

Through my work, I have observed the emotional/mental energy imbalance as being the primary cause of many health conditions and symptoms. The three most common symptoms/complaints that patients consult doctors for are: lack of energy, pain, and fear of physical and mental loss, especially the mental. As a chiropractor, I see many patients with the three aforementioned symptoms/complaints (head, neck, and back being the most common areas of pain).

Lack of vitality is caused by a decrease in the body's physical energies.

Headaches (pain in or around any part of the head) can originate from any of the emotional/mental points in or around this area, e.g. anxiety, grief, sadness, martyrdom, anger, purpose, issues with accountability, over-responsibility, betrayal, abuse, shame, hatred, jealousy/righteousness, addiction, self-worth, purpose, honour, and/or forgiveness. (See Body Charts.)

Neck pain can originate from: trust, subservience, burden, any aspect of fear, empathy and/or aspects of control.

Lower back pain (perhaps the most common form of back pain), can originate from: self-pity, respect, trust, pride, approval, hope, fear and/or over-sensitivity.

Many times, I've seen patients with recurring or chronic pain/symptoms, for which they've had treatment that was successful, but only temporarily so. With the Hale Technique, there are great outcomes when the patient is willing to accept, own, understand, and eventually forgive their part in the emotional/mental imbalance. Within a few treatments, they appear to have lasting results, for which they are very grateful, as chronic pain/discomfort leads to further symptoms relating to any of the aforementioned emotions.

The purpose of this book is to tell you what I have found in my forty plus years of investigating the human body and trying to understand how it works – and what it is trying to tell us through the display of various illnesses and symptoms.

I do not propose that I have cracked the body's true healing code, but rather from a practitioner's viewpoint how the emotional and mental energies have to be understood and in some way balanced, as they are so different and sometimes opposed to one another – causing health and behavioural issues in ourselves, our families and society in general.

As most health practitioners will tell you; we sit there and wonder why patients experience such problems/symptoms, yet clinical tests and examinations do not show evidence fitting the presenting complaint. What do I do now? If we suspect it is emotional/mental, then pills/medication/ nutrition are not always needed or effective and are sometimes refused by the patient. Suggestion of counselling/psychotherapy is often rebuked by the patient along with lifestyle changes/advice. (As I say in relation to attending a counsellor, "If you don't have any issues, there is nothing to be concerned about. What are you trying to hide?")

From my investigative testing, I find that varying forms of counselling, psychotherapy, and more latterly mindfulness techniques are very healing and helpful to people willing to co-operate and work with qualified therapists. These therapies work well towards changing the mental energies plus they have a flow-on effect into the emotional energies as well. However, over my thirty plus years of observing and testing these therapies pre- and post-sessions they appear to influence the patients' 'personal emotional' experiences but do not have any influence on 'hereditary emotions'. Addressing, understanding, and working with hereditary emotions and our individual spirituality are the key energies that promote people to find their true worth and purpose in this lifetime experience. Imbalance can and often does lead to unexplained symptoms, illness, and behavioural variances.

Various energies that are effectively influenced in treatment are:
- Chiropractic, Osteopathy – physical and spiritual energies (especially if neck and cranial (skull) treatments are included), personal, emotional energies if Neuro Emotional Technique (NET) is used.
- Acupuncture – physical and personal emotions.
- Mind therapies – mental and personal emotions.
- Massage – physical, personal emotions and often spiritual energies, especially if neck and cranium are included.
- Homeopathy – physical, personal emotions, and spiritual energies, especially if ultra-high potencies are administered.

The Hale Technique is a way of addressing these unbalanced body energies. I do not propose it is the only way but nevertheless it is an effective way to help heal the body by addressing and balancing the PEMS[1] energies. Hopefully, from my findings, other methods and techniques will be developed by others in the future that simulate similar healing outcomes.

I guess my findings can be summed up by Maureen Rose's words to me in earlier days when I would contact her for advice on a patient who was not responding to or stabilising with my treatment. She would say, "Find a technique to shut their mental mind down – they are chaotic, victims, etc. Then get into their emotional energies and correct them; It's all emotional, Bryan." She would then tell me what to look for as she could tell spiritually (God[2]-given talent). Most often the patient would phone or text back within a few days, thanking me – stating that the pain or problem was relieved within minutes to hours later. These results changed my understanding and approach to healthcare and the possibilities of providing a wider and more effective way of helping patients heal, own their lives, and grow as an individual in this chosen lifetime.

I hope and trust that patients and practitioners will have learned something new from reading this book.

---

1   'PEMS' refers to the Physical, Emotional, Mental, and Spiritual energies.
2   Wherever 'God' is mentioned the idea of a divine being or creator is meant (with respect to all beliefs).

CHAPTER 26

In conclusion
(as Bryan)

What am I doing writing a book? Actually, I have really enjoyed writing, exploring, and collecting information. My previous experience with books is that I only read to gain information; never would I consider reading for pleasure or relaxation.

In hindsight, I consider myself a very privileged man to have encountered such great teachers, mentors, patients, and supporters in my life. Many times, I have been challenged by members of my family, my circle of friends, and my patients to look at my behaviour and decisions and how they may affect other people in my life. Humility and gracefulness are values I still struggle with, but the older I get the challenges somehow become easier to accept.

My purpose of fulfilment is to learn from my patients and while I now consult patients only two days a week there is never a day that I don't come away with new knowledge and new challenges, both professionally and personally. Retirement is not an option in my life as I now realise that I have passion in my purpose, which is to experiment with my patients as to how their body works, acts and reacts – an ongoing study. My patients benefit from new treatment protocols, my associates learn more and are able to help their patients with more effective treatments and support, and I feel fulfilled from learning and contributing more.

When I started this journey of learning and development I initially became very confused, frustrated, and resentful because somehow, I instinctively knew that there was more to supporting patients' and my own health than to treat for symptom-relief only. In my early days, I was often heard to say, "I don't know why I go to work to treat patients; they all die anyway." And, "Why have I been given all this information? Give it to someone who has a better and more inquiring mind than me."

The answers eventually came to me: "You're not here to save people; you are here to help them in their journey of life." And: "Why shouldn't it be you getting this information? You chose your journey, so get on with it!" I now understand that I chose these challenges in my life. The Universe has kindly supplied me with the challenges and from fronting up, I have been rewarded.

Throughout the journey of developing and experiencing the Hale Technique, I observe that my mental and emotional health has improved greatly. I can now say that over the last ten to fifteen years I am happier, healthier and more 'at peace' with myself, my life, and my surroundings than I have ever been at any stage of my life this far. As a result, my physical health, in proportion to my age, previous physical abuses, and hereditary factors, has also greatly improved and I now feel 'in control' of my health and life in general.

Experiencing my true reality, without any embellishment, I wake up every morning and look forward to a full day of challenges, learning, and fun. I am never disappointed! At the end of most of my days I look forward to getting to bed and resting my mind and my body so that I can wake up the next day to experience more excitement and challenges. In the morning and again at the end of each day, I thank the Universe and everyone in my life who supports me to this end.

Occasionally I have a bad day. This is normal in most people's lives as it gives us balance and creates challenges, contrasting lightness with darkness. Don't dwell on it; it is just a rare bad day!

Having had a life history of melancholy and struggling with the choice of life versus death for over thirty years I now realise that although this condition occasionally still shows its ugly existence in me, I now understand that along with my gift of 'knowing', melancholy has always been my friend and moderator. **It stops me from becoming arrogant in my life's teachings!** If my melancholic condition persists, I now have a good source of treatment and help to balance my energies and health by consulting a colleague who is trained in the Hale Technique. What a gift to myself and others.

Many of my patients I have known and treated for over thirty years. We have a lifetime of learning and life experiences that we have shared together as we have grown in wisdom! They will often ask, in a genuine way, "Bryan, how are you doing?" My standard answer is that **"I am happy in my misery."** This reply always initiates laughter and further discussion. Everyone has their issues and problems in living their lives; I am no exception as I still have daily challenges in all areas of my life.

Through acceptance of my behaviour, both past and present, I have grown and been coached to understand myself and others. My healing is still ongoing and will be to the day I die as I learn to experience forgiveness of myself and others. Because of this personal journey I am not only **happy** in my life, but I have also learned to become **at peace with myself**.

I can honestly say that there is not anything much that I really want or need in my life that I do not already have. Sure, materialistic things like a new car, boat or bike are all nice but after a day or so the novelty wears off. I don't really need them; I just want them.

I have completed most of my bucket list as the further I travelled with personal development, treatment, understanding and forgiveness, the more I realised that the less I needed and wanted. I used to be like some people I hear say, "Every day above ground is a bonus" or "Enjoy every day as it could be your last." Now I enjoy my life because of the challenge I have created to learn and understand myself, the people around me, and most of all, the wonderful meaning of experiencing life itself. What a wonderful gift and opportunity we, as human beings have been given to experience, learn and grow as a human being.

One last exercise I suggest for some of my patients to test their level of true happiness and self-worth:

- Look in the mirror, just your face, after washing it and tidying your hair.
- Concentrate on looking into your eyes (the mirror of your spiritual soul).
- Don't concentrate on any pimples, imperfections, state of your hair, lack of make-up or facial symmetry.

- What do you see? A good person, someone you love to see in the mirror. A person you like, a person you can trust, and a person you respect?
- If any of those questions you cannot honestly answer yes to – you need to work on yourself.
- Babies and small children can usually answer yes to those questions. They will look at themselves and smile, giggle and talk to that person they love to see in the mirror.
- Why can't you do it?
- Try it for up to thirty seconds. It seems a long time but keep doing it until you can smile at yourself and agree it is the nicest and most honest, reliable, trustworthy, respected, and liked face you have ever known.

Twenty years ago, I hated what I saw in the mirror; now I look forward to seeing my smiling face every morning as I welcome my great day to come.

Try it. It does take time and effort but it is truly worth it, as it helps heal your past and expose your true spirituality.

Thus, the title of this book:

"Reflections on Health. In our nakedness; who are we?"

Bibliography

Merck Manual (2006). *The Merck Manual, Eighteenth Edition.* New Jersey: Merck Research Laboratories.

O'Malley, J. (1998). *The Impact of the Subluxation Model on Perception, A Cross-Cultural Study of Hilot and Chiropractic.* Victoria: Royal Melbourne Institute of Technology University.

World Health Organization. (2017). *Depression* (Fact Sheet No.369). Retrieved from http://www.who.int/entity/mediacentre/factsheets/fs369/en/index.html

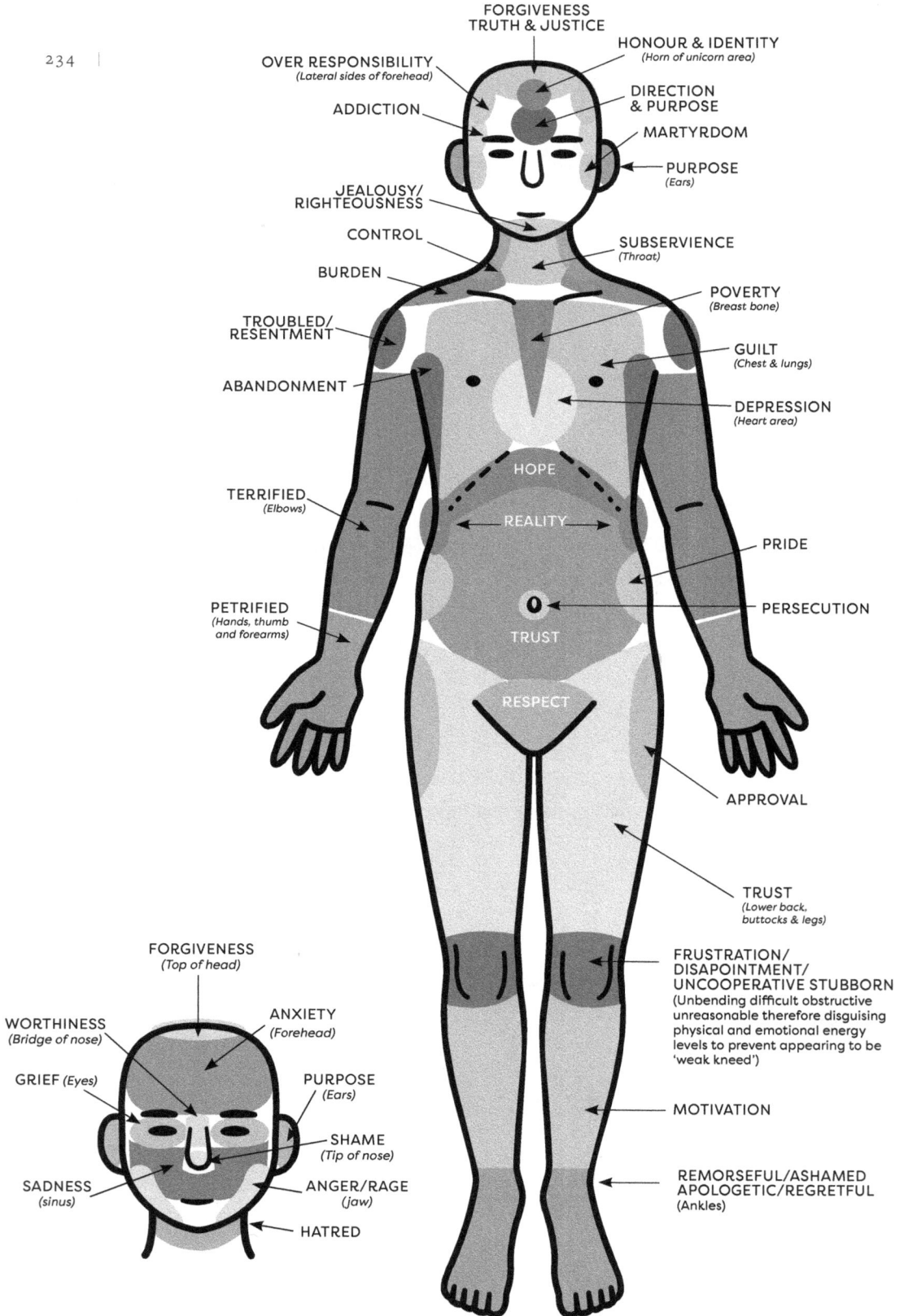

FORGIVENESS TRUTH & JUSTICE

OVER RESPONSIBILITY
(Lateral sides of forehead)

HONOUR & IDENTITY
(Horn of unicorn area)

ADDICTION

DIRECTION & PURPOSE

MARTYRDOM

PURPOSE
(Ears)

JEALOUSY/ RIGHTEOUSNESS

CONTROL

SUBSERVIENCE
(Throat)

BURDEN

POVERTY
(Breast bone)

TROUBLED/ RESENTMENT

ABANDONMENT

GUILT
(Chest & lungs)

DEPRESSION
(Heart area)

HOPE

TERRIFIED
(Elbows)

REALITY

PRIDE

PETRIFIED
(Hands, thumb and forearms)

PERSECUTION

TRUST

RESPECT

APPROVAL

TRUST
(Lower back, buttocks & legs)

FRUSTRATION/ DISAPOINTMENT/ UNCOOPERATIVE STUBBORN
(Unbending difficult obstructive unreasonable therefore disguising physical and emotional energy levels to prevent appearing to be 'weak kneed')

MOTIVATION

REMORSEFUL/ASHAMED APOLOGETIC/REGRETFUL
(Ankles)

FORGIVENESS
(Top of head)

WORTHINESS
(Bridge of nose)

ANXIETY
(Forehead)

GRIEF *(Eyes)*

PURPOSE
(Ears)

SHAME
(Tip of nose)

SADNESS
(sinus)

ANGER/RAGE
(jaw)

HATRED

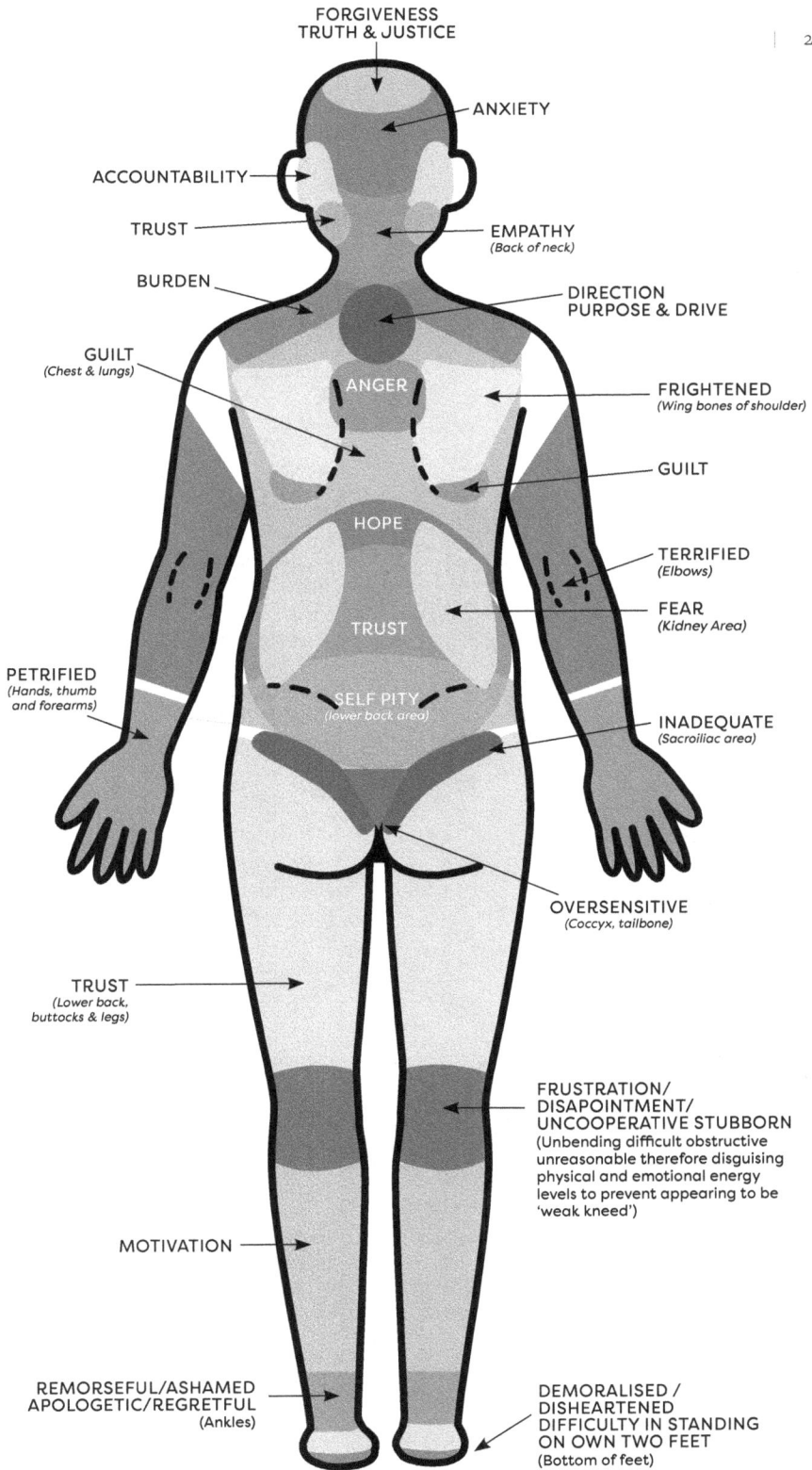

FORGIVENESS
TRUTH & JUSTICE

ANXIETY

ACCOUNTABILITY

TRUST

EMPATHY
(Back of neck)

BURDEN

DIRECTION
PURPOSE & DRIVE

GUILT
(Chest & lungs)

ANGER

FRIGHTENED
(Wing bones of shoulder)

GUILT

HOPE

TERRIFIED
(Elbows)

FEAR
(Kidney Area)

TRUST

PETRIFIED
(Hands, thumb
and forearms)

SELF PITY
(lower back area)

INADEQUATE
(Sacroiliac area)

OVERSENSITIVE
(Coccyx, tailbone)

TRUST
(Lower back,
buttocks & legs)

FRUSTRATION/
DISAPOINTMENT/
UNCOOPERATIVE STUBBORN
(Unbending difficult obstructive
unreasonable therefore disguising
physical and emotional energy
levels to prevent appearing to be
'weak kneed')

MOTIVATION

REMORSEFUL/ASHAMED
APOLOGETIC/REGRETFUL
(Ankles)

DEMORALISED /
DISHEARTENED
DIFFICULTY IN STANDING
ON OWN TWO FEET
(Bottom of feet)

Index

A

Abandonment 75
Abuse 76, 141
Accountability 77, 144
Addiction 81, 145
Agitation 68
Anger 67, 83
Anxiety 84, 146, 157, 160, 164
Applied Kinesiology (AK) 37
Approval 85, 146
Attitude 148

B

Barriers to happiness 203
Betrayal 133
Body-Mind balance 35
Born Leaders 207
Bullying 211
Burden 88

C

Case History
  Annabelle 26
  Anthony 147
  Fiona 103
  George 110
  Harold 78
  Holly 86
  Jennifer 25
  Kevin 98
  Lucy 222
  Maude 123
  Mrs T 65
  Nick 184
  Pete 27
  Sean 166
  Thomas 129
  Trevor 119
Chaos 133
Character 136
Charisma 23
Control 88
Criticised 68

D

Deal, Dr Sheldon 38
Depression 89, 148, 157, 160, 164

E

Emotions 57, 75, 205
Empathy 90

F

Facilitators 207, 209
Fate 200
Fear 69, 91
  of success 175, 177
Forgiveness 96, 213
Fretfulness 68
Frightened 92
Fury 67

G

Goals
  Personal 201
  Realistic 200
Grief 98
Guilt 100

H

Happiness
  barriers to 203
Hatred 101
Healing Model 193
Hope 102

I

Instincts 53
Intentionality 23

J

Jealousy 68, 103

Index

K

Karma 200

L

Lawlessness 68
Leadership 207
Life purpose 195
Love 61
  In Love 63

M

Martyr 106
Martyrdom 149
Melancholy 157, 164

N

Neuro Emotional Technique (NET) 38

O

O'Hagan, Brian 39
O'Malley, Dr John 38
Over-responsibility 108

P

Peacefulness 219
Persecution 112, 150
Personality 136
Petrified 94
Placebo 23
Poverty 113
Pride 114
Protégés 207, 210
Purpose
  Life 195
  True 197
  Useful 195

R

Rage 67, 83
Reality 114, 151
Respect 116
Righteousness 117, 152
Rose, Maureen 39

S

Sacro Occipital Technique (SOT) 38
Sadness 118
Self-forgiveness 214
Self-pity 119
Shame 121
Sorrow 121
Spiritual 179
Stress 171
Subservience 122, 153
Success
  fear of 175, 177
Supporter 207, 210

T

Terrified 93
The mental mind 137
Therapy and Practice Identity 23
Troubled 126
Trust 129, 154

V

Values 55
Victim 207, 211

W

Woodsford, Robin 39
Worth 131
  Materialistic 154
  Self 155
Wronged 67

HEALTHY CHOICES LEAD TO HEALTHY LIVES AND EXPERIENCES

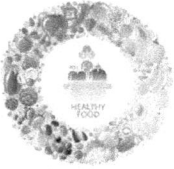

EAT A RAINBOW DIET

Lots of fresh natural foods, fruits, nuts, meat, fish, grains, and vegetables with lots of colour. Food from fast-food outlets is convenient and easy but is not always healthy. One such meal per week is okay. Sugar (especially white sugar) is a major health hazard.

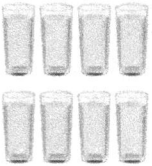

DRINKING WATER

Drink at least 6 glasses a day and filtered where possible. Tea and coffee dehydrate the body. Fizzy drinks, pop or diet pop are not healthy choices.

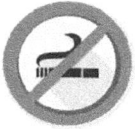

STOP SMOKING

Smoking tobacco is perhaps the most detrimental thing you can insult your body with.

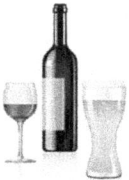

DAILY ALCOHOL CONSUMPTION

Wine, beer or spirits are also detrimental to health even if it is 1 glass per day. Red wine contains beneficial antioxidants, however the negatives of alcohol outweigh these benefits. Alcohol depresses your whole system, including your immune system. (An occasional social drink is not an issue.)

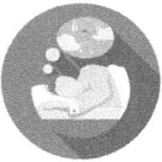

ADEQUATE REST AND SLEEP

These are essential to our body's healing powers. It is generally accepted that a minimum of 7-8 hours sleep daily is the optimum. Take time out to rest through the day even if it is sitting down for 10 minutes to take a breather. Don't eat or drink on the run; sit down to eat meals.

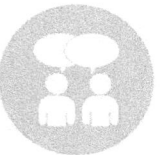

COMMUNICATION

Make an attempt to keep up with friends and family regularly. Communication is the key to healthy relationships and the solving of 'broken-down' situations. They don't contact you for the reasons you don't contact them. Take the initiative.

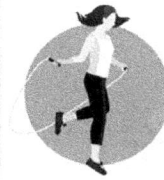

DAILY EXERCISE IS IMPORTANT

Use it or lose it. Use the stairs instead of the elevator, walk to and from the various daily chores or jobs you do throughout the day. You will feel better about yourself through doing daily exercise of a more physical nature (such as going to the gym, walking, running, cycling, swimming, yoga, etc.)

Through exercise you will improve your circulation, lymphatic drainage, and eliminate toxins through sweat. But the biggest advantage is that you will improve your mind through releasing endorphins (feel-good chemicals) within the brain. Therefore choose an exercise that you like doing and vary where and when you do it to keep you interested. Benefits of exercise are one-half physical and one-half mental.

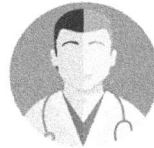

ASK YOUR DOCTOR QUESTIONS

People who understand what's going on experience less anxiety. We are here to help and, like you, we are just human too. Working in health we have either experienced your situation or have advised patients on such issues. Understanding leads to acceptance, from which we can choose forgiveness and eventual healing.

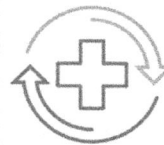

REGULAR MAINTENANCE CARE

Integrated Health suggests 2-to-6 monthly check ups to promote health and healing through balancing Physical, Mental, Emotional, and Spiritual Energies.

www.ingramcontent.com/pod-product-compliance
Lightning Source LLC
Chambersburg PA
CBHW081358270326
41930CB00015B/3342